Pain in Childbearing

Key Issues in Management

Edited by

Margaret Yerby MSc RN RM ADM C&G730 PGCEA

Senior Lecturer (Midwifery), Wolfson Institute of Health Sciences, Thames Valley
University, London, UK

Foreword by

Lesley Page BA MSc SRN SCM RNT RMT

The Queen Charlotte's Professor of Midwifery Practice, The Centre for Midwifery Practice,
Thames Valley University; The Hammersmith Hospitals NHS Trust, London, UK

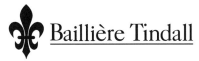

Baillière Tindall

EDINBURGH LONDON NEW YORK PHILADELPHIA ST LOUIS SYDNEY TORONTO 2000

BAILLIÈRE TINDALL
An imprint of Harcourt Publishers Limited

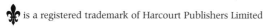
First published 2000

ISBN 0 7020 2299 3

British Library Cataloguing in Publication Data
A catalogue record for this book is available from the British Library

Library of Congress Cataloging in Publication Data
A catalog record for this book is available from the Library of Congress

Note
Medical knowledge is constantly changing. As new information becomes available,
changes in treatment, procedures, equipment and the use of drugs become necessary.
The author and the publishers have, as far as it is possible, taken care to ensure that
the information given in this text is accurate and up to date. However, readers are
strongly advised to confirm that the information, especially with regard to drug usage,
complies with the latest legislation and standards of practice.

The
publisher's
policy is to use
**paper manufactured
from sustainable forests**

Printed in China

Contents

Contributors

Carmel Bagness MA RGN RM ADM PGCEA
Programme Leader (Midwifery), Wolfson Institute of Health Sciences,
Thames Valley University, Slough, Berkshire, UK

Maureen Boyle MSc RN RM ADM PGCEA
Senior Lecturer (Midwifery), Wolfson Institute of Health Sciences, Thames
Valley University, London, UK

Helen Crafter MSc RGN RM FPCert ADM PGCEA
Senior Lecturer (Midwifery), Wolfson Institute of Health Sciences, Thames
Valley University, London, UK

Christine Grabowska BSc MSc Lic Ac RN RM ADM PGCEA
Senior Lecturer, Wolfson Institute of Health Sciences, Thames Valley
University, London, UK

Sarah Keeble BSc(Hons) RGN RSCN ENB405 998 870
Clinical Nurse Manager, Neonatal Intensive Care Unit, Chelsea and
Westminster Hospital, London, UK

Jancis M Shepherd RGN RM ADM PGCEA MTD
Senior Lecturer (Midwifery), Wolfson Institute of Health Sciences, Thames
Valley University, Slough, Berkshire, UK

Caroline Squire MSc Lic Ac RM ADM PGCEA
Senior Lecturer, Wolfson Institute of Health Sciences, Thames Valley
University, London, UK

Raewyn Twaddle RSCN ENB405
Sister, Neonatal Intensive Care Unit, Chelsea and Westminster Hospital,
London, UK

Margaret Yerby MSc RN RM ADM C&G730 PGCEA
Senior Lecturer (Midwifery), Wolfson Institute of Health Sciences, Thames
Valley University, London, UK

Foreword

Is the pain of birth no more than an intense form of toothache to be relieved at all costs? Why do some women 'remember' that the pain of labour was excruciating yet consider the experience to have been 'hard work but wonderful'? Why are some women traumatized by the memory of the pain of birth, so that they would never go through labour again? When and how does the unborn or newborn baby feel pain, and is this pain likely to forge memories for the life to come? Why have we overlooked the pain that women often experience in the postnatal period, especially when we know it adds distress in a time of upheaval and exhaustion? Midwives and doctors in the maternity services face such questions every day of their working lives.

The opportunity for the complete relief of the pain of labour, through epidural anaesthesia, has provided us with a fundamental dilemma. Is it as unreasonable to expect a woman to endure the pain of labour without an epidural as it would be to expect someone to go to the dentist and have a filling without a local anaesthetic – or is there more to it than that?

Pain in Childbearing helps us consider these questions thoughtfully and on a basis of sound information. To answer them we need to understand not only the physiology and psychology of pain, and the pharmacology of pain relief, but also the way culture and beliefs about birth affect our perceptions of pain. This book provides plenty of information in these areas; but, perhaps above all, it makes clear the importance of the personal support of midwives in educating and being 'with women' in labour. It also provides detailed advice and discussion on non-pharmacological ways of comforting women and reducing the pain of labour. Moreover, we are left in no doubt about the importance of providing comfort and pain relief to the woman in the postnatal period, and of relieving any suffering experienced by the baby.

Recently I have watched with concern the rapid rate of increase in the uptake of epidurals. There is a cost: at a minimum we see it in the increase in the rate of operative deliveries associated with the procedure; but there is more to it than that. Not only does the most severe pain of human experience usually accompany birth, but also great joy. The birth of the baby is the start of new life, the formation of a family, and when all is well the start of the love affair between mother and baby and the father that is the foundation of secure, healthy, loving life. our aim should be, as this book describes clearly, to help women move away from a passive acceptance of either simply enduring pain or having the pain taken away. Women have different needs and give birth in different circumstances. Some women in some circumstances do need pain relief in labour. But, when women are given adequate personal support, fewer take up the option of pharmacological pain relief. The increasing confidence given by personal support, the reduction of fear and the encouragement of the body's natural opiates can help the majority of women – help them not only to survive labour and birth but also to see it as a wonderful experience, remembering the pain through the joyful euphoria of those early moments of the baby's life. In childbirth, agony often gies way to ecstasy!

Pain in Childbearing avoids extreme positions, offering careful and sensitive arguments and information. It is humane in its emphasis on the relief of suffering, not only for the mother but also for the baby. Any midwife or doctor reading this book will be encouraged to see birth as far more than a toothache to be relieved and to see that there are a number of ways to help women cope with the pain and hard work of labour.

Ultimately we should aim to leave women with the feeling 'I did it myself, now I can cope with anything – even the tribulations (and joys) of years of parenthood!' The key to this sense of achievement is threaded in clear themes throughout many of the chapters. It requires giving women an active role, providing effective, sensitive, personal support and the offer of simple comfort measures such as massage, while knowing when pharmacological pain relief is needed. Every professional involved in the care of childbearing women should read this book.

Lesley Page

Introduction

This book is the culmination of ideas derived from my Master's thesis, and is intended as a gift to students who struggle with the aetiology of pain. While my particular area of interest is the physiology of pain and its pharmacological relief, the contributions of my co-authors have resulted in a comprehensive review of pain associated with childbirth. Its contents bring together a range of pertinent issues regarding pain in a single volume and convenient format to enable the student to be better informed and thus be more effective when with women in childbirth.

The antenatal pain chapter concentrates on symphysis pubis dysfunction, a condition that has gone unrecognized for many years yet creates persistent pain and disability through and beyond the childbearing period. It covers aspects of assistance required by the mother in labour and subsequently on her return home.

The physiology of pain is approached by discussing uterine contractions and the nerve supply to the uterus and the cervix, and how pain might be created by the labour process. The physiological effects of the process of labour and pain on the mother and fetus are viewed from the perspective of the body balancing its vital functions when put under stress. Finally the chapter discusses pain research.

The psychology chapter poses a number of questions which are, hopefully, answered. For example, why is physiological process so painful for many women? Does pain in labour have a purpose? Other aspects in this chapter include the role of support and the attitudes of the health professional to pain in labour.

Alternative and pharmacological methods of pain relief discuss both invasive and non-invasive mechanisms by which pain can be eased or near totally removed. Alternative therapies include the power of touch, and the use of hypnosis and guided imagery. Most importantly, they include the ability of women to feel in control, giving them a sense of self-worth and achievement in coping with their pain. Not all women are able to cope with the pain of labour in a natural way and the use of pharmacological medications helps them to overcome fear and pain in labour. These interventions are not without side-effects on both the mother and the fetus.

The use of drugs and various interventions in the course of a woman's labour has moral and legal issues, especially those relating to a midwife's practice. The importance of informed choice for women in labour must not be forgotten or devalued and this is discussed in Chapter 6.

Postnatal pain, apart from 'after pains', sometimes comes as a surprise for women and receives little sympathy from midwives. The many causes of pain and thus loss of the sense of well-being in the postnatal period have been examined, and these include headache, and breast and perineal pain.

No book of this kind is complete without including the historical perspectives of pain and its relief in childbirth. A step back in time reviews the developments and advances that altered practices within midwifery over the years. The chapter on socio-cultural aspects of pain includes the influences of modern technology on pain relief, culture and stereotyping.

In the concluding chapters, pain in the fetus and neonate are discussed, and the development of the nervous system, pain reflexes and pain sensation of the fetus in utero is traced. Once born and adapting to the extrauterine environment, the neonate will experience pain and this alters the neonate's physiological response. There is a need for all carers to improve their ability to assess how much pain the neonate is experiencing by the use of appropriate assessment tools and then to use and analgesic that is effective, if this is felt necessary.

In writing this book, my co-authors and I hope to stimulate in students a spirit of enquiry that encourages them to seek and continue to learn throughout their lives.

London 1999

Margaret Yerby

Acknowledgements

I would like to thank my colleagues who helped me to make my interest a reality by their contributions.

To Felicity Plaat, Brian Allen and Dave Croker who were expert readers on Chapters 3 and 8: thank you for your expert opinions.

Thank you to my family and friends who proofread my chapters and supported me throughout the project.

1

Pain relief: past and present

Caroline Squire

INTRODUCTION

The desire for pain relief in labour has been in existence in most societies for as long as human experiences have been recorded. This chapter is an overview of pain-relieving methods past and present, omitting contemporary non-pharmacological methods such as the use of water and acupuncture. As such, western attitudes towards pain will be touched upon as a theme throughout as well as the growth of women's groups and their relationships with obstetricians and midwives. Emphasis is placed on the history from the early years of this century to the present day.

Historically, a vast array of concoctions have been reported in the literature, not just to relieve pain in labour, but, more commonly, to expedite labour. The use of opiates and herbs, such as hemp and mandrake, was mentioned in early Chinese writings, the drinking of wine was noted in Persian literature, and wine, beer and brandy were commonly self administered in Europe during the Middle Ages (Dickersin 1989). In ancient Egypt, pain-relieving solutions, such as incense, wine and groundup scarab beetle or tortoise shells, were applied externally to the lower abdomen (Chamberlain 1993). Zerubhabel Endecott, a seventeenth-century physician of Salem, Massachusetts, recommended for 'sharp and difficult travel in women with child' a mixture of powdered virgin's hair and fried ant's eggs in the milk of a red cow! (Moir 1980).

Moir reveals that brutal force could be used to expedite birth as well and describes how Apache squaws were sometimes suspended from a tree by a rope under their arms. Braves would then grasp the woman above the uterus and swing against it. Women in the Serang Islands gave birth, at times, standing and bound to a tree by the arms held above the head (Moir 1980).

Mauriceau (1697) prescribed bleeding, a well-used remedy of the time:

> If a woman be plethorick, it may be convenient to bleed her a little; for by this means, her breast being disengaged, and her respirations free, she will have more strength to bear down her pains, which she may do without danger.

More usefully, he continues with some very helpful advice:

> The weak woman should be strengthened, the better to support her pains, giving her good Jelly-Broths, with a little wine and a toast in it . . . If she fears the pains, let her be comforted, assuring her that she will not endure many more, but she be speedily delivered.

Some of these methods may have been of some benefit, particularly the use of opiates and hemp, but largely the relief of pain would have been achieved through peer support, notably from other women. Kitzinger (1992) writes of women in Elizabethan times being supported by God Sibs, 'sisters in God' who orchestrated everything that took place in the birthing room and were resented by men who gradually changed their name to the pernicious word 'gossip'. Vincent-Priya (1992) describes how Aborigine women go to the women's camp to give birth with their mothers and other female relatives. Cherokee women give birth with four women, either family, friends or neighbours at home but where all male relatives except their husbands are excluded:

> Reassurance, massage and emotional support are the methods which traditional midwives use to relieve pain (Vincent-Priya 1992).

Jordan (1993) has written concerning Mayan women in Yucatan, Mexico. Here she describes how mothers may travel long distances to be with their daughters and their husbands during birth. If labour seems prolonged, then other women afford extra support be they friends or relatives:

> Jointly and by turns, they give the woman mental and physical support. They encourage her, urge her on, and sometimes scold her, always letting

her know that she is not alone, that the business of getting this baby born will get done.

ATTITUDES

Historically, pain was characterized as an affective feeling state rather than a sensation (Craig 1994). Pain could be attributed to evil spirits or witches and incantations and charms were used for its relief. In traditional societies such practices continue, though they may relate to non-problematical births and the delivery of healthy children as well. In rural Sri Lanka, McGilvray (1982) describes how the childbirth house is shuttered and closed during the actual delivery to protect the mother and baby from evil spirits, ghosts and demons who are attracted to the blood and contamination. Labouring women carry an iron object on them at all times as an antidemonic safeguard. Vincent-Priya (1992) reveals many instances of the supernatural being invoked or appeased during births. She met a traditional Malay midwife who prayed over a glass of coconut water so that her guiding spirit was infused into it. This was given to the labouring woman who, therefore, took in the spirit to help her give birth. Many midwives in current practice have experienced bottles of holy water on the bedside cabinet in the delivery room or prayers being said by orthodox Christians or Muslims. These rituals may be enacted to protect the mother and child and, as a form of support, may have pain-relieving effects as well.

To the ancient Greeks pain was considered an essential emotional component of the human spirit, the negative counterpart of pleasure which should be avoided like sadness or bitterness; but it was not considered a sense like hearing or sight. This notion was not to change until Descartes' concept of pain in the seventeenth century, when he proposed that the sensory nerves conduct non-corporeal copies of the objects perceived to the brain. This was the beginnings of the concept of mind–body dualism which is referred to in Chapter 5. The argument as to whether pain should be construed as an emotion or sensation continued until the rapid advances of biomedicine in the nineteenth and twentieth centuries. Until then, pain was considered an emotional state.

When considering pain as an emotional state, it is possible to understand how, during the Middle Ages, explanations of pain were underpinned by the biblical notion that physical suffering during birth is a punishment of womankind for Eve's temptation of Adam (Genesis chapter 3: verses 13–16). As Mauriceau (1697) writes concerning the pain of childbirth:

Most people believe that there is no other reason for the cause of this evil, but because God hath so ordained it, and that woman, according to his word, must bring forth with pain because of her sin, according to what is written in the third chapter of Genesis: I will greatly multiply thy sorrow and conception; in sorrow thou shalt bring forth children and thy desire shall be to thy husband.

Traditionally, midwives drew heavily on their empirical knowledge of herbs, foods, poultices, rituals and good luck charms, but such departure from religious doctrine was considered as blasphemy and many were condemned as witches and heretics (Ehrenreich & English 1973, Simkin 1989). The same fate might occur to women who sought help from traditional midwives. Moir (1980) describes how Euphame MacCalzean was burned at the stake in Edinburgh, without mercy of previous strangling. She had sought the aid of a 'witch' to ease her labour pains onto a dog which ran away and was never seen again.

Within this approach of universally shared responsibility for original sin is the related explanation of personal responsibility for pain. Both share the belief of pain as punishment and Dickersin (1989) informs us that radical medical groups, such as the hydropaths in the nineteenth century, believed that obstetric pain was a direct result of leading an 'unnatural' life, as no natural process is painful if individuals lead healthy lives (whatever that meant). In our contemporary industrialized society, to be healthy means we have to be slim, take daily exercise and eat nutritious food. It is easy to participate in the notion of 'victim blaming' (Crawford 1977) if an individual seems not to take individual responsibility for their health and may be obese, smoke or enjoy a diet full of carbohydrate. Perhaps as midwives we need to be careful not to 'victim blame' women in labour. Many midwives will have heard colleagues say to women who are finding labour very painful and who seem unprepared: 'Didn't you attend parentcraft classes?', as if parent education was the ultimate analgesia. The attitude is judgemental viewing the woman as deviant and ignorant which is not so far from the attitude of the hydropaths.

Simkin (1989) cites Caton (1985) to describe a new age of enlightenment during the Renaissance where pain and suffering were no longer passively accepted as the result of sin, although this notion continued beyond the separation of the relationship between the Church and medicine. Pain was now seen to be destructive and the pursuit of pleasure and absence of pain became desirable and both morally and medically acceptable. Medicine as a profession emerged by separating itself from the Church and the barber's trade and burgeoned throughout the eighteenth and nineteenth centuries in the age of scientific discovery.

PHARMACOLOGICAL ANALGESIA

The first obstetric anaesthetic was administered by Young Simpson of Edinburgh on 19 January 1847 in the form of ether. This was soon superseded by chloroform which was first employed, again by Young Simpson, on 8 November 1847 (Moir 1982b). For the next 100 years, ether, chloroform and, later, nitrous oxide remained almost the sole anaesthetic agents in use in obstetrics. Chloroform was dropped onto an open mask or handkerchief with each contraction but had the unfortunate side-effect of causing respiratory depression in the baby, atonic postpartum haemorrhage, irregularities of the heart and liver damage (Chamberlain 1993).

Chloroform was the most effective anaesthetic of its time. However there was much opposition for its use in childbirth, although it was considered suitable for surgery and dentistry. Some of the opposition came from the Church for reasons outlined earlier in the chapter. Young Simpson considered that the quotation from Genesis (chapter 3: verse 16), 'in sorrow shalt thou bring forth child', was actually a mistranslation of the Hebrew and the crucial word at issue should have been translated as effort or stress rather than sorrow. In addition, some doctors disagreed, stating that pain is even desirable during surgery and childbirth:

> *Pain is to the mother safety; its absence a destruction. Yet there are those bold enough to administer the vapour of ether or chloroform even at this critical junction forgetting it has been ordered that in sorrow shall she bring forth. (Chamberlain 1993: p 4).*

John Snow, renowned as an epidemiologist with regard to typhoid, was greatly influenced by Simpson and, as a physician, administered chloroform to Queen Victoria for the birth of her eighth child, Prince Leopold, in 1853. Such was the success, he used it again for her ninth and tenth births. Many authors have considered that this royal seal of approval led to its greater acceptance (Moir 1982a, Dickersin 1989, Chamberlain 1993), but Connor & Connor (1996) disagree. In their historical review they state that although some members of the public did know of Queen Victoria's use of chloroform, the fact was largely ignored by the lay newspapers, and comments in the medical press remained antagonistic. Furthermore, there was no proportionate increase in the obstetric anaesthetic practice of John Snow following her use of chloroform.

Twilight Sleep

In the early years of the twentieth century, experimentation in obstetric anaesthesia took place. In 1902, Von Steinbuchel of Germany introduced the combination of scopolamine hydrobromide and morphine sulphate. The former blunts the memory and the latter is a powerful hypnotic and pain reliever. Together, they induce continuous sleep with lack of memory so that women were unable to recall the events of labour. They caused respiratory depression in their babies however. The use of 'Twilight Sleep' spread rapidly, although it was limited by the fact that a doctor had to be in attendance. It was best administered on an individual basis but because of the workloads of midwives and obstetricians, attempts were made to use standardized protocols. These were less successful (Chamberlain 1993).

Twilight Sleep initiated some of the first organized social movements of women. In the USA, the National Twilight Sleep Association (TWA) was formed to combat the predominantly male obstetric profession. Their mission was to inform women that 'modern science has abolished that primal sentence of the scriptures upon womankind' (De Haven Pitcock & Clark 1992). Interestingly, this group of women changed obstetric practice and its relationship to pharmacological methods of pain relief profoundly. First, one of the drawbacks of Twilight Sleep was the problem of the labouring woman who might, unknown to her, thrash about so wildly as to hurt herself. It was necessary, therefore, to have women monitored closely throughout labour and to restrain them if necessary. Clearly, there was an issue of safety here and the TWA lobbied forcefully to move birth from home to hospital, and for the hospital to provide padded beds, special restraining gowns and protective helmets! Second, it brought to centre stage the issue of control of the birthing process (De Haven Pitcock & Clark 1992).

Inhalational analgesia

Nitrous oxide was used widely in general surgery and dentistry in the nineteenth century but was not used in obstetrics until the 1930s. In 1933, R.J. Minnitt, a Liverpool anaesthetist, designed his apparatus for the administration of nitrous oxide and air (Moir 1982b). Originally, the concentrations were 45% nitrous oxide and 55% air but this was later altered to 50% of each (Chamberlain 1993). In 1936, the Central Midwives Board (CMB) approved the use of the Minnitt apparatus and it was used until its withdrawal in April 1970. According to Moir (1982b) this marked the end of an era of hypoxic analgesia. In 1965, following CMB approval, nitrous oxide was administered premixed with oxygen via the Entonox apparatus and by the Lucy Baldwin apparatus.

Trichlorethylene (Trilene) is related to chloroform but less toxic and, although used by obstetricians since 1941, it was not approved by the CMB until 1955 (Moir 1982b). It was administered via the Emotril Automatic and the Tecota Mark 6 apparatus. Generally, analgesic effects took longer than nitrous oxide and oxygen but the effects lasted for longer. In 1983, the CMB withdrew its approval for independent midwives and it is not used now.

Methoxyflurane (Penthrane) was introduced in 1959 and quite widely used in obstetrics in the USA. Midwives were permitted to use 0.35% in

England in 1970 administered via the Cardiff inhaler. Concern was voiced concerning Penthrane and possible adverse effects on renal function, although it was never demonstrated after intermittent inhalational analgesia in labour (Moir 1980).

Needless to say, the CMB laid down specific instructions as to the use of inhalational analgesia. A general comment can be observed in Myles (1964):

> *To be successful, instruction during the prenatal period is essential for when feeling nervous on her admission to hospital, distracted with pain or stupefied by drugs, the woman cannot comprehend the directions given her.*

One can appreciate the maternalistic tone of the quotation though it was meant kindly.

Various other drugs were used during the first half of the twentieth century, including narcotics, barbiturates and other sedatives, tranquillizers and amnesiacs administered separately or in combination in a variety of ways, i.e. by inhalation, orally, intravenously, intramuscularly, rectally. The sedative drugs that midwives could give are listed in Box 1.1 (Myles 1964). Those drugs which had to be ordered by the doctor are listed in Box 1.2.

Box 1.1 Sedative drugs that midwives could give

◆ Chloral hydrate
◆ Potassium bromide
◆ Syrup of chloral
◆ Welldorm tablets
◆ Trichloryl tablets
◆ Pethidine
◆ Pethilorfan
◆ Tincture of opium
◆ Trichloryl syrup

Box 1.2 Drugs which had to be ordered by the doctor

◆ Morphia
◆ Heroin
◆ Omnopon

Pharmacological analgesia

Pethidine was developed in 1939 in Germany and became extremely popular as a strong analgesic for wounded troops in the Second World War. It is a powerful antispasmodic but the evidence concerning its efficacy as an analgesic is far from clear. It may be that its soporific effects have been confused with analgesia and the overwhelming majority of prospective trials continue to report that pethidine is, at best, a poor analgesic in labour (Scrutton 1997). Originally, it was not a controlled drug and many people, often women for the treatment of dysmenorrhoea, became addicted in the late 1940s. In 1949, pethidine was brought under the Dangerous Drugs Act and its use strictly regulated. It is now one of the most commonly used drugs throughout the west, although its popularity is waning, probably due to the rise of the epidural and its side-effects as a respiratory depressant on the baby (see Ch. 8).

Morphia was not extensively used in labour, apart from the historical use of opiates as mentioned previously, until the introduction of Twilight Sleep. It went out of favour because women felt nauseated and the babies were born respiratorily depressed. Currently, morphia is rarely used except in the narcotics administered with epidurals.

Regional analgesia

Spinal subarachnoid analgesia was accidentally produced by Corning in 1885 in USA. His technique was unreliable and Quincke in 1891 improved the technique of the procedure of lumbar puncture. However, Bier of Germany became the first doctor to use spinal analgesia for surgery. Apparently, pain relief was achieved but patients suffered greatly from headaches and vomiting which were caused, in the opinion of Moir (1980), by the use of unsterile tap water to dissolve the cocaine crystals and the free leakage of cerebrospinal fluid.

Over the past 20 years, regional techniques of analgesia and anaesthesia have emerged as the major approach to pain relief in childbirth, not only for vaginal and operative vaginal births but for caesarean section as well. Paracervical blocks were popular in the 1950s and early 1960s, particularly in France, Germany, USA and Scandinavia, but are rarely used now as a result of reports of fetal bradycardia, acidosis and even death.

Caudal epidural blocks have been supplanted by lumbar epidural blocks because, with the former, larger volumes of anaesthetic were needed to produce adequate pain relief which resulted in more blocked spinal segments and it was possible for the anaesthetist to miss the caudal canal and insert the needle into the baby's scalp resulting in death when the anaesthetic was administered (Dickersin 1989). Recent advances include lumbar epidural for use in labour, spinal anaesthesia for use at caesarean section, combined spinal epidural blocks and, most recently, the use of patient-controlled epidural analgesia. The uses and side-effects will be explored in Chapter 8 and the consideration of the epidural as part of the medicalization of childbirth will be discussed in Chapter 5.

THE INFLUENCES OF CAMPAIGNS FOR ANALGESIA BY WOMEN

In the years between the wars, there was an influential campaign led by women such as Lady Baldwin to find a method of analgesia that could be used by midwives. The reason for this was so that women who gave birth at home, regardless of socioeconomic circumstances, could have some form of analgesia administered to them. At that time, most births were at home and, prior to the inception of the National Health Service in 1948, families had to pay for the services of a midwife or general practitioner (GP). Midwives, of course, were cheaper but were not allowed to administer chloroform which was the most commonly used drug. GPs administered chloroform and, therefore, its use was restricted to the middle classes who could afford such services. With the introduction of nitrous oxide and air, later oxygen, the campaign seemed to have found the answer. However, as Beinart (1990) comments citing the Royal College of Obstetricians and Population Investigation Committee (RCOG/PIC 1948), their aspirations were ill founded because the provision of such analgesia varied very much from one area to another and it was particularly poor with regard to women giving birth at home as opposed to hospital or nursing home.

In 1928, the National Birthday Trust Fund was set up, spearheaded by another group of upper-class women as a result of concern over the high maternal mortality rate (Beinart 1990). It managed to raise substantial funds and began to seek ways of extending analgesia for all women. For example, it funded the development of the Minnitt apparatus previously described. Midwives, upper-class women and obstetricians seemed to be in accord with one another at this time. The introduction of analgesia which midwives could use clearly broadened their expertise, while obstetricians were unable to provide analgesia themselves for all women. GPs were reluctant because much of their maternity practice at home and in nursing homes depended on their exclusive abilities to administer chloroform (Beinart 1990). This probably marked the decline in the GP obstetrician which, of course, accelerated after the Peel Report in 1970 which made provision for 100% hospital births. This move from home to hospital also marked the decline of the midwife and the ascendancy of the obstetrician.

NATURAL CHILDBIRTH

At the same time as the Twilight Sleep debate and the call for analgesia for all, another approach to pain relief was developing. Grantly Dick Read was a young doctor when he attended the birth of an impoverished woman in Whitechapel. She was the first woman to refuse his offer of chloroform (see Ch. 4).

This left a great impression in his mind:

Civilisation and culture have brought influences to bear upon the minds of women which have introduced justifiable fears and anxieties concerning labour. The more cultured the races of the earth have become, so much more dogmatic have they been in pronouncing childbirth to be a painful and dangerous ordeal (Dick Read 1943: p 9).

Parent education was central to the natural childbirth movement, with labour interpreted as work rather than suffering and active participation in labour and birth encouraged. Clearly, this was the antithesis of Twilight Sleep. The notion of women being in control, however, should be seen in the context of the age. From Dick Read's case histories, a high degree of paternalism and control was evident:

Mrs ... had her baby yesterday afternoon. She had not been a satisfactory patient and throughout her pregnancy, there had been a great tendency to know everything.

Further on in her labour, she appeared to be finding labour difficult:

I had to be strict with her, and told her that there were times when we did not expect a woman to play the fool; this was a serious thing; she was to do as she was told and would meet with very little difficulty (Dick Read 1943: p 187).

In 1956, the National Childbirth Trust (NCT) was established under the name of the Natural Childbirth Association and today is the largest supportive group for mothers in the UK. Prunella Briance, the founder, formed the organization to promote the ideas of Dick Read (Kitzinger 1990). By 1959, it began to shift from Dick Read's philosophy to Lamaze's theory of prepared childbirth. This theory, termed 'psychoprophylaxis' was pioneered by Velvosky and Nicolaiev in the 1920s and 1930s and was based, loosely, on Pavlov's work on conditioning. It was thought that fear generated unfavourable reflexes but the brain, correctly programmed, could distract the pain reflex by a series of breathing exercises which would then minimize pressure of the diaphragm on the uterus (De Haven Pitcock & Clark 1992).

Lamaze visited Nicolaiev's clinic in Leningrad in 1951 and used the technique, culturally adapted and with elements of Dick Read's philosophy, in France. It soon crossed the Channel and the Atlantic to become the most famous technique for women who wanted drug-free labours in the 1960s. Kitzinger (1990) informs us that while Dick Read's theory promoted the idea that a woman should submit to her uterus and surrender to nature, Lamaze's philosophy was one of victory over the body rather than surrender.

Initially, the NCT shared the medical view that most women did not know what was best for them (Kitzinger 1990). Erna Wright, a follower of Lamaze, wrote a postscript for professionals which begins:

I sincerely hope that the way in which this book is written has not annoyed you (Wright 1968: p 239).

Currently, this view has changed and a woman's right to make her own decisions is central to the NCT's philosophy.

The NCT and the Association for Improvements in Maternity Services (AIMS) were both founded in the 1950s and they remain strong today. The next 30 years also saw the development of organizations such as the Active Birth Movement, the Society to Support Home Confinements and Maternity Alliance (Durward & Evans 1990). Their strength probably lies in being lay movements, outside the culture of biomedicine and the NHS Bureaucracy, although consumers with experience.

Leboyer published his book *Birth without Violence* in 1977, which gave insight into a new consciousness regarding the baby's experience of birth. Unfortunately, this became known as the 'Leboyer' method which had its merits for many women in terms of peace and quietness with darkened rooms but tended to focus on the fetus to the exclusion of the mother (Odent 1982). Michel Odent began to publish widely in the 1970s and 1980s concerning his birthing philosophy that is practised in Pithiviers, France. He and his colleagues believe in a woman's ability to give birth absolutely and thus create surroundings in which she is undisturbed. Here, pain relief is absent except for the rare caesarean birth and he has noticed that in unmedicated births women seem to forget themselves and what is happening around them.

Arney & Neill (1982) consider that obstetrics as a profession has used pain relief to control women. They argue that the natural childbirth movement sought to enable women to consider and experience pain as their own pain, the pain that accompanies active participation in attempts to master a challenge. They feel that obstetricians felt alienated because of their loss of control and regrouped themselves by ensuring that women were closely monitored under the guise of support so that women, in effect, were persuaded that they would experience pain without that support. Thus, it became disempowering:

> *Women seized pain from obstetricians and, for a short moment made it their own. But then, with extraordinary rapidity, obstetrics mobilised 'a rush of knowledge' to analyse this new aspect of childbirth. Joined by social scientists who modelled the quality of childbirth experiences, obstetrics recaptured pain, relocated it so that it stood outside women, in between them and the optimal childbirth experience which could be achieved only with obstetricians' managerial assistance (Arney & Neill 1982).*

This point of view may be difficult to understand when we have been enculturated into a biomedical framework in terms of education and environment. Perhaps the quest for control over pain by women can be seen in the trend towards the use of complementary, non-pharmacological methods and these will be considered in Chapter 7. Suffice to say that most women today want the right to make decisions and be informed about their births including, clearly, options concerning pain and its relief in labour.

CONCLUSION

Today, the issues surrounding control of pain remain prevalent. Are women in control of childbirth the less they feel? Is the notion of working *with* pain lost in our technological age? When we support women, do we really monitor them and, thus, disempower them? Is the epidural the best of all worlds – no pain but full consciousness? To conclude, should we be concerned by an article in *The Times* in which Professor Fisk argues that natural childbirth is a risky business and women should be given the option of an elective caesarean section:

> *It's much safer than driving a car (Corrigan 1997).*

This would, of course, obviate the need for consideration of pain in labour but would that mean women were really in control, or are the sensations of labour something to work with, respect and even cherish?

ANNOTATED BIBLIOGRAPHY

Fordham M, Dunn V 1994 Alongside the person in pain. In: Holistic care and nursing practice. Baillière Tindall. London, especially ch 5, p 75

This chapter refers to nursing practice and the management of pain but I think it is useful for midwives to consider some of the issues. For example, there are sections concerning partnership in pain, problem solving and individualized care which are particularly relevant to midwifery.

Ginesi L, Niescierowicz R 1998 Neuroendocrinology and birth 1: stress. British Journal of Midwifery 6: 659–663

This article is written by lecturers in human biology who are also National Childbirth teachers. The areas discussed concern a new perspective of the subtle and dynamic hormonal balance that may develop during physiological labour. They note remarkable similarities between the changes and behaviour of the birthing women and those of other sexual responses. They feel that their paper adds weight to the body of evidence which suggests that creating a calm, safe environment for the birthing woman is vitally important.

Niven CA 1992 Psychological care for families. Butterworth Heinemann, London, especially ch 2, p 40

This is a very useful book written by a psychologist who is also a nurse. This chapter considers stress and anxiety in childbirth, pain and preparation for childbirth, coping and social support in childbirth as well as the father's experiences. She draws from international literature and a particularly interesting section is to be found on page 47 when she considers that duration of labour is not always negatively correlated with the intensity of pain overall.

Niven C 1994 Coping with labour pain: the midwife's role. In: Robinson S, Thomson AM (eds) Midwives, research and childbirth, vol 3. Chapman & Hall, London, ch 5, p 91

This is a very interesting chapter in an edited book in which the author describes her research study which was part of a larger study on factors affecting labour pain. In this chapter, Dr Niven considers pain assessment measures as well as the methodology used in her research. The latter includes the assessment of the effects of obstetric factors such as parity, induction and duration of labour, weight of the baby, and the effects of psychological factors such as the desirability of the pregnancy, expectations of childbirth, antenatal education and the presence of the partner during labour, on pain perception.

Porter J 1997 Psychological methods of pain relief. In: Reynolds F, Russell R, Scrutton M, Porter J (eds) Pain relief in labour. BMJ Publishing Group, London, ch 2

Dr Porter is an anaesthetist and writes a useful chapter concerning psychological methods of pain relief. She divides her chapter into four sections. The first section concerns preparation for labour and she considers preparation for 'natural' childbirth, psychoprophylaxis, antenatal preparation in the 1990s, mechanism of action, efficacy, complications and disadvantages. The second section concerns support during labour and the author considers the roles of the midwife, partner and doula and looks at the efficacy and implications of such support. The third section considers hypnosis and the author looks at its efficacy, effect on labour, mechanism of action, effects on the baby, and the disadvantages and complications. The fourth section considers biofeedback and, again, looks at efficacy and disadvantages of this kind of psychological method of pain relief.

REFERENCES

Arney W, Neill J 1982 The location of pain in childbirth: natural childbirth and the transformation of obstetrics. Sociology of Health and Illness (1): 1–24

Beinart J 1990 Obstetric analgesia and childbirth. In: Garcia J et al (eds) The politics of maternity care. Clarendon Press, Oxford, ch 6, pp 118, 123

Caton D 1985 The secularization of pain. Anaesthesiology 62: 493-501

Chamberlain G 1993 The history of pain relief in labour. In: Chamberlain G, Wraight A, Steer P (eds) Pain and its relief in labour. Churchill Livingstone, London, ch 1, pp 1, 4, 5

Connor H, Connor T 1996 Did the use of chloroform by Queen Victoria influence its acceptance in obstetric practice? Anaesthesia 51: 955–957

Corrigan S 1997 The benefits of having a nice, clean cut. *The Times, News International* 15 July, p 16

Craig KD 1994 Emotional aspects of pain. In: Wall P, Melzack R (eds) Textbook of pain. Churchill Livingstone, London, ch 12, p 220

Crawford R 1977 You are dangerous to your health. International Journal of Health Services 7: 663–680

De Haven Pitcock C, Clark RB 1992 From Fanny to Fernand: the development of consumerism in pain control during the birth process. American Journal of Obstetrics and Gynaecology 167: 581–587

Dickersin K 1989 Pharmacological control of pain during labour. In: Enkin et al (eds) Effective care in pregnancy and childbirth. Oxford University Press, Oxford, ch 57, pp 913, 936

Dick Read G 1943 Childbirth without fear, 2nd edn. William Heinemann, London, pp 5, 9

Durward L, Evans R 1990 Pressure groups and maternity care. In: Garcia J et al (eds) The politics of maternity care. Clarendon Press, Oxford, p 257

Ehrenreich B, English D 1973 Witches, midwives and nurses: a history of women as healers. The Feminist Press, New York

Jordan B 1993 Birth in four cultures, 4th edn. Waveland Press, Prospect Heights, Illinois, p 33

Kitzinger J 1990 Strategies of the early childbirth movement. A case-study of the National Childbirth Trust. In: Garcia J et al (eds) The politics of maternity care. Clarendon Press, Oxford, pp 92, 107, 109

Kitzinger S 1992 Ourselves as mothers. Doubleday, London, pp 96, 107, 109

Leboyer F 1977 Birth without violence. Fontana Fletcher & Son, Norwich

Mauriceau F 1697 The diseases of women with child and in child-bed. Andrew Bell, London, pp 145, 146

McGilvray DB 1982 Sexual power and fertility in Sri Lanka. In: MacCormack C (ed) Ethnography of fertility and birth. Academic Press, London, ch 2, p 58

Moir D 1980 Obstetric anaesthesia and analgesia, 2nd edn. Baillière Tindall, London, pp 1, 4, 6

Moir D 1982a Pain relief in labour. Churchill Livingstone, London

Moir D 1982b Pain relief in labour. Churchill Livingstone, London, pp 1, 4, 5

Myles M 1964 A textbook for midwives. Churchill Livingstone, London, pp 262, 263, 268

Odent M 1982 Birth reborn. Souvenir, London, p 12

Royal College of Obstetricians & Gynaecologists and Population Investigation Committee 1948 Maternity in Great Britain. Oxford University Press, Oxford

Scrutton M 1997 Systemic opioid analgesia. In: Reynolds F (ed) Pain relief in labour. BMJ Publishing Group, London, ch 5

Simkin P 1989 Non-pharmacological methods of pain relief during labour. In: Enkin M, Keirse JNC, Chalmers I (eds) Effective care in pregnancy and childbirth. Oxford University Press, Oxford, ch 56, p 894

Vincent-Priya J 1992 Birth traditions. Element, Shaftesbury, pp 68–70, 82, 89

Wright E 1968 The new childbirth. Tandem Books, London, p 239

2

Symphysis pubis dysfunction*

Jancis Shepherd

INTRODUCTION

Symphysis pubis dysfunction (SPD) is the term used to describe the pain, instability and limitation of mobility and functioning of the symphysis pubis joint during pregnancy and childbearing. At present many midwives and other health professionals are unaware of the condition or its longer-term effects. The disabling and debilitating nature of SPD is often unrecognized. Health professionals may fail to appreciate that the woman may experience difficulty in trying to care for her family, infant feeding problems, social isolation, depression or relationship difficulties. How the mother with SPD is affected both physically and emotionally in the weeks and months following childbirth is unacknowledged.

As a midwife is the health care professional most likely to give continuity of care during pregnancy, labour or the puerperium (Department of Health 1993), it is essential that she has the skills to recognize SPD and offer

---

* The basis of this chapter is taken from Shepherd J, Fry D. Symphysis pubis pain. Midwives 1996; 109 (1302): 199–201. Material used is reproduced with the kind permission of *Midwives.*

17

appropriate advice on its management. The midwife needs to understand how SPD affects the woman both physically and emotionally, so that she may offer advice, information and moral support.

Symphysis pubis dysfunction describes the symptoms of pain, pelvic instability and joint dysfunction experienced by the woman. Traditionally where joint separation of greater than 10 mm has been apparent the condition has been referred to as symphysis pubis diastasis, symphysiolosis or separation of the symphysis pubis joint. However, pain, instability and dysfunction of the joint can occur with joint laxity rather than a demonstrable separation, thus the term symphysis pubis dysfunction is used.

Snelling in 1870 described the condition thus:

> *The affection appears to consist of relaxation of the pelvic articulations, becoming apparent suddenly after parturition or gradually during pregnancy, and permitting a degree of mobility of the pelvic bones which effectively hinders locomotion and gives rise to the most peculiar, distressing and alarming sensations.*

It has recently been acknowledged that this is an under-recognized and underdiagnosed condition (Taylor & Sonson 1986, Scriven et al 1991, 1995). Many health professionals are unable to give optimum care as they are unaware of how it manifests or how disabling and debilitating the condition can be. At best the symptoms may resolve in weeks or months, at worst long-term morbidity may necessitate surgical fixation of the symphysis pubis.

INCIDENCE

The incidence is variously reported as ranging from one case in 300 (Kubitz & Goodlin 1986) to one in 20 000 (Eastman & Hellman 1966) occurring in primigravidae and multigravidae. These incidences are given where separation of the joint has been confirmed, rather than the broader definition of dysfunction, which describes the symptoms experienced by the woman. The incidence is greater where the latter criterion is used.

PHYSIOLOGY OF SYMPHYSIS PUBIS DYSFUNCTION

The onset of symptoms may be insidious in the second or third trimester, may be linked to a specific activity, or arise during or after delivery.

Essentially symptoms are caused by instability of the symphysis pubis joint. In the non-pregnant state, the circumferential envelope of ligaments at the joint, especially the inferior ligament, neutralizes the shearing forces on the joint allowing only minimal movement during activity. As the function of the pelvis is to transfer body weight to the legs all pelvic joints must be stable; any dysfunction in one joint will be reflected in the functioning of the others.

To prepare the pelvis for delivery of the fetus, the pregnancy hormones cause the collagen content of the ligament to be altered. The ligament becomes more extensible, resulting in increased movement of the joint, therefore causing potential instability. This occurs especially in the ligaments of the sacroiliac joints and symphysis pubis. The normal 4-mm gap between the bone ends of the symphysis pubis may asymptomatically increase to as much as 9 mm (Grieve 1976) during pregnancy. It is also thought that enzymes, causing resorption of bone, contribute to the widening of the symphysis particularly in the third trimester (Gamble et al 1986). Although the increased separation regresses shortly after delivery (Lindsey et al 1988), complete reversal of laxity in the pelvic joints may take 3–5 months in all postpartum women.

The male and female symphysis pubis undergoes natural degenerative changes throughout the lifecycle (Gamble et al 1986). In the female, bony changes are evident in the symphysis pubis whether the woman miscarries or carries the pregnancy to term. Putschar (1976) states that the delivery of an infant of greater than 2.3 kg will always result in traumatic damage in the symphysis pubis joint, causing it to be permanently more vulnerable to the normal weight-bearing stresses. If instability caused by a long-term diastasis persists, the natural degenerative changes in the joint will occur sooner in life leading to chronic pain.

A diagram of the pelvis is given in Figure 2.1 and symptoms experienced with SPD are listed in Box 2.1.

Box 2.1 Some symptoms that may be experienced with SPD

◆ Mild to severe groin/pubic pain that is increased by weight bearing, this may radiate to the medial aspect of the upper thigh(s). This may be described as a burning pain or bruised sensation in the symphysis pubis

◆ A 'waddling' gait, 'dragging' of a leg

◆ An audible or palpable 'click' and/or 'crunching' sensation felt in the joint

◆ Low back pain

◆ Pain on movements that involve standing on one leg such as dressing, getting in and out of the bath, climbing the stairs or movement in bed

◆ Pain on any activity that involves parting or lifting the legs such as reaching to open a window, getting in and out of the car, sexual intercourse

◆ Pain on lifting and carrying any weight, e.g. baby, toddler, car seat, shopping

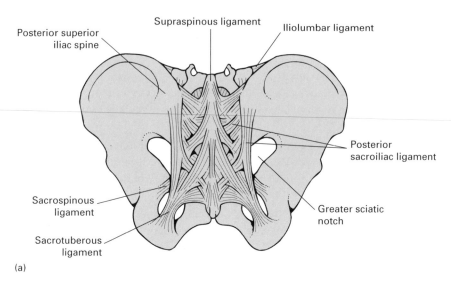

Posterior superior iliac spine
Supraspinous ligament
Iliolumbar ligament
Posterior sacroiliac ligament
Sacrospinous ligament
Greater sciatic notch
Sacrotuberous ligament
(a)

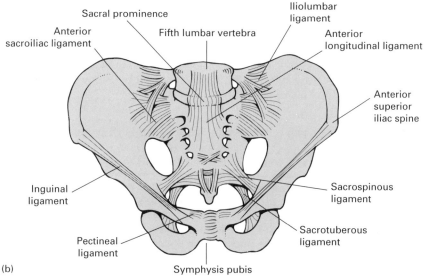

Sacral prominence
Anterior sacroiliac ligament
Fifth lumbar vertebra
Iliolumbar ligament
Anterior longitudinal ligament
Anterior superior iliac spine
Inguinal ligament
Sacrospinous ligament
Pectineal ligament
Sacrotuberous ligament
(b)
Symphysis pubis

Figure 2.1 The pelvis: (a) posterior view; (b) anterior view.

It is not uncommon for explanations for these symptoms to include 'aches and pains' of pregnancy, round ligament strain or urinary tract infection. Although the midwife should be alert for these conditions, they do not lead to the pain and limitation of function previously described.

Although it has been accepted in the literature that a separation of the symphysis pubis joint of less than 10 mm is asymptomatic but a diastasis of 10 mm or more will be symptomatic (Lindsey et al 1988), it is the authors' experience that a woman can be symptomatic yet not have a demonstrable diastasis if an X-ray is taken postnatally. Thus the term SPD is used to describe the symptoms experienced by the woman.

If confirmation of a diastasis is sought, ultrasound scanning using a 7.5-Mhz transducer (Scriven et al 1995) offers a simple, relatively pain free, procedure that does not involve ionizing radiation. Although confirmation does not aid the management of the condition, it may aid any future follow up of the client. Currently X-ray examination is unlikely to be performed to avoid irradiation of the gonads.

The traditional reasons given in the literature for diastasis mainly relate to trauma: precipitous labour, difficult instrumental delivery, excessive forced abduction of the hips. Cephalopelvic disproportion, previous or existing pelvic abnormality and multiparity are also recognized (Lindsey et al 1988). Where trauma at delivery is involved symphysial pain becomes apparent to the woman immediately. As labour management has improved these causes are less likely to be seen in current practice.

There appear to be two groups of women who do not fit the traditional causes. In one group the symptoms are unrecognized antenatally and therefore midwifery management cannot take account of the potential problems. Retrospectively the women will acknowledge that symptoms were present antenatally and delivery has exacerbated them. In the second group no symptoms manifest antenatally but appear postnatally, with a variable time of onset. Women who have had uncomplicated, spontaneous vaginal deliveries of average weight babies have reported symptoms 12–24 hours postpartum. The reasons for this are unclear. However, Driessen (1987) noted a similar later onset (1–2 days) in his small survey in Malawi and postulated that this was due to gradual swelling within the joint, which could account for the delay in onset. This highlights the need for the midwife to be alert for women who complain of unusually severe pain with difficulty in mobilizing postnatally that is not attributable to perineal pain.

MANAGEMENT OF SYMPHYSIS PUBIS DYSFUNCTION

The aim is to limit stress on the pelvic joints and reduce pain levels. It is important to advise and encourage the woman to rest the symphysis pubis joint as much as possible, this means ceasing non-essential activities and accepting offers of help with housework, other children and shopping. She should avoid prolonged weight bearing, climbing the stairs, standing on one leg (e.g. when dressing) and twisting movements of her back. It is essential that she avoids abducting her hips and keeps her legs as close together as is comfortable in activities such as getting in and out of a car and turning in bed. When resting, placing a pillow between the legs and keeping the knees in apposition may be beneficial. If a shower is available this is less traumatic to use than a bath.

A clear explanation to both the woman and her partner of the condition and its management is vital. The explanation should avoid the use of alarming words, for example 'split', 'separated' or 'broken' pelvis (ACPWH (Association of Chartered Physiotherapists in Women's Health) 1996), the emphasis on pelvic joint laxity being preferable and less frightening.

The foregoing advice and change in lifestyle can be difficult and frustrating for some women to follow; however, experience has shown that when the woman complies, symptoms can be noticeably reduced. If symptoms do not subside appreciably with this advice the woman should be referred by her doctor to a physiotherapist, ideally one who is experienced in obstetrics. A full pelvic and back assessment should be undertaken. As symptoms warrant, a pelvic support such as tubigrip worn as in Figure 2.2 or 2.3 (McIntosh 1995), a trochanteric belt or symphysis pubis support may give relief of pain. Where weight bearing is painful the use of elbow crutches will maintain mobility while reducing strain on the pelvis. Appropriate analgesia should be offered and prescribed.

A plan of management needs to be formulated for care during labour. This will require good communication between all members of the team caring for the woman both antenatally and postnatally.

Care during labour

The woman and her labour partner will need to be aware of suitable positions for the different stages of labour. Involvement and clear information about

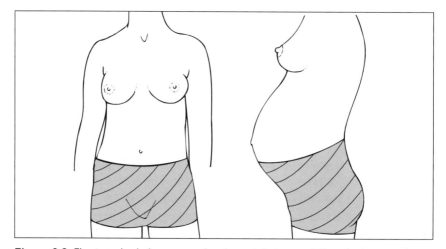

Figure 2.2 Elasticated tubular support bandage tripled around ilium (redrawn with permission from McIntosh 1995).

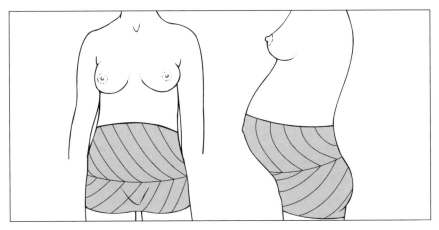

Figure 2.3 Elasticated tubular support bandage doubled around upper abdomen and tripled around symphysis pubis (redrawn with permission from McIntosh 1995).

the forthcoming labour may help to reduce the fear and anxiety that the expectant mother may experience. Reassurance that adequate pain relief is available, if needed, should be given. In severe cases elective caesarean section may be undertaken.

Where vaginal delivery is anticipated the range of hip abduction should be assessed prior to labour (McIntosh 1993). Attempts should be made to ensure that the woman is not placed in any position that is outside her range of pain-free hip movement. Finding a position of comfort for the labouring mother may be difficult as her mobility can be severely limited. For some women being upright and mobile within their capabilities may help them to cope with labour. A lateral position may be preferable for vaginal examination. The midwife needs to be aware that epidural or spinal anaesthesia, although offering valuable pain relief, could mask the symptoms of symphysis pubis pain and allow excessive mobilization of the joint, leading to increased pain postpartum. Where epidural/spinal anaesthesia is required the midwife should ensure that the woman's range of pain-free hip abduction is not exceeded while the anaesthesia is effective. The partner's assistance may be required to keep her legs adducted during this time.

For the second stage of labour a lateral position or a supported 'all fours' position will reduce strain on the symphysis pubis. If the lithotomy position is needed for a forceps delivery or Ventouse extraction, the hips should be abducted simultaneously for as short a time as possible. Extreme pain is likely throughout the procedure. Ideally, vaginal examination, forceps delivery and suturing would be undertaken in a lateral position. The midwife should be aware that forced abduction of the hips as in the woman pushing with her feet upon the midwives' hips could lead to SPD. This may not be defensible practice if subsequent litigation arises.

Care in the postnatal period

Postnatal management of the condition is very similar to antenatal management. Referral to a physiotherapist will be necessary for assessment and advice. However, the mother will require complete bedrest and all physical care from the midwife for 24–48 hours, until acute pain subsides. The assessment of risk factors that predispose to deep vein thrombosis should be undertaken, TED stockings should be worn while on bedrest and thromboprophylaxis initiated if appropriate. Ankle exercises may help to prevent deep vein thrombosis.

Assistance will be needed with personal hygiene including taking the woman to the toilet in a wheelchair and instructing her not to sit astride the bidet. The midwife will need to help the mother with the baby's care, handing the baby to the mother for cuddles and giving help with feeding and changing. A comfortable position will need to be found for breastfeeding and assistance given with correct positioning. Mobilization within her own capability, with the aid of elbow crutches if necessary, is then encouraged to gradually increase her activities. Analgesia will be given as required, a pelvic support may give relief. Pain levels will be her guide to how much weight bearing she can undertake.

Transfer home

Whether transfer home occurs antenatally or postnatally the home circumstances need careful review. The proximity of the bathroom, number of stairs, help available from the partner, family and friends will be required. The mother may need to stay at home for some days or weeks postnatally. Substantial help in caring for the new baby and other children may be required. Where elbow crutches are being used to alleviate pain this limits all other activities as both arms are used to walk. The mother may be unable to lift or carry her new baby, needing the baby handed to her for feeding. Carrying the baby downstairs may be impractical because of pain, and the fear of falling or dropping the baby. Changing or bathing the baby may only be possible if a surface at waist height is available. Using a pram as a changing surface may be a practical solution. Where the mother is unable to walk or to drive, her dependence upon family or friends for social activities, shopping and taking siblings to playgroup or school increases. Assistance may be needed with household tasks such as loading and unloading the washing machine or dishwasher, ironing and cleaning. Activities that involve forward flexion and rotation of the hips, such as pushing a vacuum cleaner or floor mop, may provoke extreme pain. The mother may feel very inadequate in caring for her family and experience social isolation or relationship difficulties. It is possible that these factors may increase the likelihood of depression occurring. Assistance in the home may need to be sought from social services. An occupational therapist may be able to give advice on energy conservation and planning daily activities to limit pain. Aids such as a bath board may be available to enable the woman to manage more comfortably. A 'helping hand' gadget may be supplied to pick up items from the floor.

When the mother does feel able to resume her routine she can be advised that the weight of a baby in a carry sling may provoke pain and should be avoided. Placing the car seat in the car and then strapping the baby into it is more practical than attempting to lift the baby in the seat. Many supermarkets now offer designated mother and baby car parking that can be used antenatally and postnatally. If asked, supermarkets may provide an assistant to push the shopping trolley, pack bags and load them into the car. Some shops are now offering telephone shopping and local delivery. If this is available this would enable the mother to feel less dependent on friends and relatives.

RECOVERY

Whether the condition occurs antenatally, during labour or postnatally, a very clear explanation of the condition, treatment and prognosis will be needed by the woman and her partner. The recovery period is variable, from weeks to months (Lindsey et al 1988), and may be years in extreme cases (Scriven et al 1995). To date, experience has shown that pain-relieving modalities, for example ultrasound, make no difference to pain levels. With severe chronic cases surgical fixation may be required to stabilize the joint. Women should be warned that even when symptoms have subsided symphysial pain may be felt premenstrually, if so activities that are known to exacerbate the symptoms should be avoided.

Further research is required to determine why some women are more susceptible than others to severe pelvic instability, and which form of management has the least morbidity. The use of alternative therapies in the management of pain is at present unevaluated. Data is required to evaluate the likelihood of recurrence in subsequent pregnancies, and if so, which mode of delivery is advisable.

It is the authors' experience that where health professionals' knowledge of symphysial pain is increased, the postnatal incidence is markedly reduced. In women presenting with antenatal onset of symptoms, morbidity appears to be decreased where advice is followed.

CONCLUSION

It is essential to redress the current situation of the lack of awareness of the condition among health professionals. Because the prevailing attitude is either one of disbelief of the symptoms or a lack of sympathy (McIntosh

1993), and an inability to give information about this 'rare' condition, the sufferer may feel extremely isolated. The early recognition and management of the condition by the midwife will not only improve the quality of life for the sufferer but also may help to reduce morbidity in the longer term. The midwife needs to be able to offer optimum care, visiting until 28 days postnatally if necessary before transferring care to the health visitor. During this time the midwife may need to refer the woman to the appropriate health professionals and utilize the services of voluntary agencies.

Reflective scenario 2.1

Amanda and Robert are expecting their third baby. They live in a semidetached house in a community that has a post office, a mini market and a chemist. Robert spends a lot of time away on business; they have no family living locally. Nicola, who is 3 years old, attends the local playgroup three mornings a week from 9.00 to 12.00 a.m. Andrew who is 6 years old attends the local school.

Amanda has a spontaneous vaginal delivery at term, David weighs 3.600 kg and is to be breastfed. They are transferred home to your care 12 hours after delivery. When you visit, Amanda complains of pain in her back and difficulty in walking. Robert is due away on business the following day.

1. What may be wrong with Amanda?
2. Devise a care plan that will meet Amanda's physical and emotional needs:
   a. for the next 48 hours
   b. for the next week.
3. What advice and information will Amanda and her family require from you?
4. Which health professionals, services and agencies may you need to enlist to assist Amanda?

Useful resources

◆ A leaflet giving advice on SPD can be obtained free by sending a stamped addressed envelope to: The Association for Chartered Physiotherapists in Women's Health (ACPWH), c/o CSP, Chartered Society of Physiotherapy, 14 Bedford Row, London, WC1R 4ED

◆ A support group for SPD is: British DSP Support Group, Mont Hamel House, Office 2, Chapel Place, Ramsgate, Kent, CT11 9RY. Tel: 01843 587356; Fax: 01483 587523

◆ HTTP://DSP.future.easyspace.com

◆ E-mail: BritishDSPSupport@compuserve.com

ANNOTATED BIBLIOGRAPHY

MacLennan AH, MacLennan SC 1997 Symptom giving pelvic girdle relaxation of pregnancy, pelvic joint syndrome and developmental dysplasia of the hip. The Norwegian Association for Women with Pelvic Girdle Relaxation (Landforeningen for Kvinner Med Bekkenlosningsplager). Acta Obstetrica et Gynecologica Scandinavica 76: 760–764

MacLennan & MacLennan, in conjunction with the Norwegian Association for Women with Pelvic Girdle Relaxation, report upon a postal survey of 1609 Norwegian women with pregnancy-initiated pelvic joint pain. This study identifies the long-term morbidity associated with the condition and the limitations of current treatment therapies. The incidence of hip dysplasia in the children of the women surveyed was five times the usual Norwegian incidence. A genetic susceptibility to joint dysfunction in mother and fetus possibly due to relaxin physiology is postulated.

Östergaard HC 1997 Lumbar back and posterior pelvic pain in pregnancy. In: Vleeming A, Mooney V, Dorman T, Snijders C, Stoeckart R (eds) Movement, stability and low back pain: the essential role of the pelvis. Churchill Livingstone, Edinburgh, ch 33, pp 411–420

Lumbar back pain, posterior pelvic pain and the epidemiology, biomechanics, diagnosis and treatment of these conditions is discussed. This text would be of interest for midwives, as pelvic instability, its detrimental effects during pregnancy and parturition and possible forms of management are clearly described.

REFERENCES

ACPWH 1996 Symphysis pubis dysfunction guidelines. ACPWH/Chartered Society of Physiotherapy, London
Department of Health 1993 Changing childbirth report. HMSO, London
Driessen F 1987 Postpartum arthropathy with unusual features. British Journal of Obstetrics and Gynaecology, 94: 870–872
Eastman NJ, Hellman LM 1966 Williams obstetrics. Appleton Century Crofts, New York, pp 820–821
Fry D 1992 Diastasis symphysis pubis. Journal of the Association of Chartered Physiotherapists in Obstetrics and Gynaecology 71: 10–13
Gamble JG, Simmons SC, Freedman M 1986 The symphysis pubis. Clinical Orthopaedics and Related Research 203: 261–272
Grieve G 1976 The sacro iliac joint. Physiotherapy 62: 384–399
Kubitz RL, Goodlin MD 1986 Symptomatic separation of the pubic symphysis. Southern Medical Journal 79(5): 578–580
Lindsey MD, Leggon R, Wright D, Nolasco D 1988 Separation of the symphysis pubis in association with childbearing. Journal of Bone and Joint Surgery 70A(2): 289–292
McIntosh JM 1993 Incidence of separated symphysis pubis. Midwives Chronicle and Nursing Notes Jan, 23
McIntosh JM 1995 Treatment note: an alternative pelvic support. Journal of the Association of Chartered Physiotherapists in Women's Health 76: 28

Putschar WGJ 1976 The structure of the human symphysis pubis with special consideration of parturition and its sequelae. American Journal of Physical Anthropology 45: 589–594

Scriven M, McKnight L, Jones D 1991 Diastasis of the symphysis pubis in pregnancy. British Medical Journal 303: 6 Jul, 56

Scriven M, McKnight L, Jones D 1995 The importance of pubic pain following childbirth: a clinical and ultrasonographic study of diastasis of the symphysis pubis. Journal of the Royal Society of Medicine 88: 28–30

Snelling FG 1870 Relaxation of the pelvic symphyses during pregnancy and parturition. American Journal of Obstetrics and Gynecology 2(4): 561–596

Taylor RN, Sonson RD 1986 Separation of the symphysis pubis: an underrecognised peripartum complication. Journal of Reproductive Medicine 31: 203–206

3

Physiology of labour pain

Margaret Yerby

INTRODUCTION

The birthing process is undoubtedly accompanied by pain for all but a few women. Pregnancy is a natural, physiological event culminating in the birth of a baby that has developed from a minute ball of cells to a new human being. It is a time of development for the fetus and adaptation for the woman both physically and psychologically. In anticipating and awaiting for labour to start there is time for both partners to prepare for the event, in particular to prepare for the experience of pain that is ultimately felt to various degrees as labour commences, advances and culminates in the birth of the baby.

Pain is very subjective and each individual will feel pain in various strengths. It is as Melzack and Wall (1991) states 'a very private experience' and only the person experiencing that pain can know how and where it is felt.

29

Whether this is created by physiological damage or the perfectly normal physiological process of labour, pain is very real to the person experiencing it. Sensitive, responsive and empathetic management is the key when supporting women through the birthing process. Women experiencing this pain on a progressive continuum may adopt their own way of dealing with the process. Some may perceive pain at the commencement of labour as intolerable, while for others pain only becomes intolerable just before the birth of the baby. Every woman is an individual and copes with labour in very different ways.

PREGNANCY CHANGES

During pregnancy women experience many changes and accept that pain will be experienced as part of the birth process. This is only part of a very complex transition from a single person to a mother with responsibilities. The birth process and the pain it creates are a psychological and physiological event, and the psychological approach to pain will alter the mother's feelings to it (Lowe 1991). Raphael-Leff (1991) describes pregnancy as a 'roller coaster' of changing emotions that, with other events, will impinge on the experience of pain. The fear, anxiety, pain cycle described by Dick Read (1950) will affect the whole process of labour and the feelings following the event will be marred by these subsequent fears. It has been suggested that women who have knowledge of birth and an understanding of the events involved will experience less pain (Kirkham 1991). In this chapter the physiology of pain will be discussed and an attempt will be made to demystify why the event which is the physiological culmination of pregnancy is such a painful one.

Women experience various discomforts during the 9 months of pregnancy. As their time approaches for giving birth an unease sets in when psychologically they prepare for labour, an event which will be painful for them. The feeling of low sacral backache, or low abdominal period-like pain, is a common feature at the beginning of labour. This is then accompanied by regular uterine contractions which increase in strength and length producing more pain that will continue until the baby is born. The ambiguity of early symptoms can create consternation, particularly the primigravid woman who is often uncertain if labour has truly started until pain increases and contractions become stronger. It may be her first experience of pain other than in a mild form, yet she may find that she is able to cope if she has developed pain-coping strategies as part of her preparation for birth through antenatal education. The primigravida will also experience on average a longer labour as the cervix takes longer to dilate in the first labour than in subsequent labours. This undoubtedly contributes to increased tiredness and exhaustion, both of which influence her perception of pain. The multiparous woman is prepared for the pain of labour; her recognition of the onset and her ability to cope with pain will be influenced by previous experience in labour or other painful events in her life. If she coped well previously and remembered labour as a good experience then pain may well be minimal (Niven & Gijspers 1984).

INFLUENCES ON UTERINE ACTIVITY–CONTRACTION AND THE COMMENCEMENT OF LABOUR

The commencement of labour is influenced by numerous factors, the maturity of the fetus and its biochemical relationships via the placenta to its mother, the position of the baby within the uterus and the softening of the cervix. Theories about the initiation of labour exist and are well substantiated by research in animals. However it is still impossible to say to any potential mother when labour will commence and give a definite time and date, unless medical intervention takes over (Goff 1993).

The uterus in the non-pregnant state contracts regularly maintaining muscle tone, but it is not until the contractions exceed a certain strength that they are felt by the woman. During the normal cyclical events of menstruation the uterus is dependent on hormonal influences from the ovary to control its activity. These hormones will continue to influence uterine activity for the duration of pregnancy, an example being the influence of progesterone which inhibits uterine contractions during implantation to enable the conceptus to cleave to the spongy uterine lining (Vander et al 1994). It is also important to maintain levels of progesterone throughout pregnancy to maintain 'uterine quiescence' (Llewellyn-Jones 1990). Research in sheep has shown that the level of progesterone is lowered by endogenous prostaglandins, this has not been proven in the case of man. If proven, it would support the hypothesis of progesterone–oestrogen ratio modification and the progesterone levels lowering, thus permitting the uterus to contract (Keele et al 1983).

During menstruation the uterus will contract forcefully to aid expulsion of the unwanted thick lining of the uterus and may be felt as low abdominal pain of variable intensity; for some women this is extremely painful. This has been associated with raised levels of prostaglandin which creates strong contractility of the uterine muscle thus inducing pain sensations. Prostaglandin $F_{2\alpha}$ is found in menstrual blood flow (Keele et al 1983) and is also found in increased amounts in the amniotic fluid before term (Austin & Short 1990). It is thought to be an important substance in the initiation of labour. Because of their contractile properties prostaglandins mobilize calcium at the cellular level within the uterine muscle, thus enhancing muscular contractility (Carston 1973). Aspirin in therapeutic doses has been shown to decrease prostaglandin synthesis by blocking cyclooxygenase, an enzyme which modifies arachidonic acid by adding oxygen to produce the prostaglandins. This may delay the onset of labour; however the small dose that may be used to prevent platelet aggregation in hypertensive disorders in pregnancy has little effect on this pathway (British National Formulary 1996).

PAIN AND LABOUR

Why should pain be of such significance in this physiological event? Like menstruation the uterus contracts in labour, the contractions increase in frequency and strength until the baby is born. The early pain felt by women in labour is similar to menstrual pain. These contractions occur regularly from the third trimester onwards and can be as strong as labour contractions and may well stimulate labour but there is no pain felt by the woman (Gibb 1993). Termed Braxton Hicks contractions, they increase their intensity towards term (Ramsey 1994). The significant difference is that in labour the lower segment of the uterus is pulled upwards, the cervix begins to efface and then dilates. Stretching disturbs soft tissues, stripping away the membranes from the cervix and causing the 'show' of early labour (Bonica & Chadwick 1990). Bonica & Chadwick (1990) cite research by Moir (1939) and Javert & Hardy (1950) that links the pain of labour directly to the stretching of the cervix and lower uterine segment. This was demonstrated when during a caesarean section under local block women experienced little discomfort when the uterus was palpated and pulled, but experienced pain similar to labour pain when the cervix or lower segments were forcefully dilated.

The processes of stretching of the cervix and stripping away of fetal membranes are associated with prostaglandins released from the fetal membranes and the maternal decidua, particularly in spontaneous labour (Fuentes et al 1996). These phenomena are not purely accidental or coincidental but are linked to physiological preparation of the body for the birth experience. Fuentes et al (1996) showed in their research on samples of amnion from labouring and non-labouring women that there was a twofold increase of cyclooxygenase, the enzyme required to produce prostaglandins, in the labouring group. The activation of this enzyme and a subsequent prostaglandin surge lends support to much earlier research reported by Mitchell et al (1977) that following a vaginal examination there was a prostaglandin F increase in peripheral blood plasma 5 minutes following the examination. This may well be why women in labour experience more pain and in some circumstances have stronger uterine contractions following vaginal examination.

Manipulation and examination of the cervix in labour may well stimulate an inflammatory process, which as well as releasing prostaglandins also stimulates the release of chemical substances that sensitize the nerve endings which stimulates the transmission of pain. The nociceptors in the cervix are sensitized by substances such as histamines, serotonin and bradykinins (Keele et al 1983). Bradykinin in particular stimulates the A and C fibres for a considerable time following the event. It could be hypothesized that repeated vaginal examinations will increase this discomfort and stimulation of pain and chemical changes which may be necessary for the progress of labour.

UTERINE NERVE SUPPLY

The autonomic nervous system serves the uterus with sympathetic and parasympathetic nerve fibres. The nerves which supply the uterus are ill defined, but nerve pathways are known (Williams et al 1989). Nerve pathways of the uterus and cervix arise from afferent fibres of the sympathetic ganglia. Nociceptive nerve endings in the uterus and cervix pass through the cervical and uterine plexuses to the pelvic plexus, the middle hypogastric plexus, the superior hypogastric plexus and then to the lumbar sympathetic nerves to eventually join the thoracic 10, 11, 12 and lumbar 1 spinal nerves (Fig. A.1). Signals are then received at the dorsal horn of the spinal column (Bonica & Chadwick 1990) and then via the spinothalamic tract to the higher centres of the brain to become a conscious pain sensation. The nerve supply to the perineum and lower pelvis from the second and third sacral nerve roots meet the plexuses from the uterus at the Lee Frankenhauser plexus at the uterovaginal junction (Stjernquist & Sjöberg 1994).

The autonomic nervous system is both inhibitory and excitatory with cell bodies in nerve ganglia as the nerve plexus mentioned above. The multiple receptors in the body of the uterus and the cervix are α_1 (excitatory) and β_2 (inhibitory) receptors which create contraction and relaxation respectively in the sympathetic system. Robinson et al (1977) cites Bhalla et al (1972) that β-adrenergic receptors stimulate cyclic adenosine monophosphate (CAMP) which inhibits myometrial activity, whereas the parasympathetic system produces a variable effect (Vander et al 1994). The functional control of the uterine smooth muscle is controlled by the autonomic nervous system (Keele et al 1983) and an interplay with hormonal substances (Williams et al 1989). Bernal & Lopez (1996) suggest that although the autonomic system may physiologically affect uterine activity it is not essential for labour, as activity has been identified in women in labour who are paraplegic or who have had sensory block with an epidural or a 'bilateral lumbar sympathectomy'. The nerve receptors in the uterus are sensitive to pressure or stretch, creating contraction of the smooth muscle of the uterus. As pressure increases tissues stretch and actual damage or potential damage occurs, releasing substances that create pain especially in the cervix which is dilating rapidly as labour progresses.

Hormone–nerve interactions

From experiments adrenergic nerves are influenced by oestrogens and progesterones. Oestrogen is found to increase the noradrenaline content of the nerve, progesterone decreases it (Stjernquist & Sjöberg 1994). The full-term uterus contracts to noradrenaline and relaxes to adrenaline (Steer 1991).

Oestrogens also stimulate the release of prostaglandins by their action on the α-adrenergic receptors (Egater & Husslein 1992). Oestrogen–progesterone ratios alter towards term and this change influences the uterine myometrium to increase the gap junctions between each individual muscle fibre. This action enables an improved communication system in the myometrium and increases the sensitivity of the muscle fibres to contractile agents (Huszar & Roberts 1982). The uterine muscle fibres need to communicate with each other to encourage coordination and the ability of the uterus to act as one. It is quite possible for smooth muscle to contract and pull in any given direction at once. It is important that the uterus contracts in a unified manner as uncoordinated uterine activity does not expel the fetus and prolongs labour and increases pain perception (Llewellyn-Jones 1990).

Receptors

All tissues contain nerve endings. Pain receptors termed nociceptors are responsible for the perception of pain from 'chemical, thermal or mechanical stimulation' (Bullock 1992). Pain commencing in the uterus and cervix will become painful depending on the woman's pain threshold and the psychological influences at the commencement of labour (Whipple 1990). In labour the nociceptors in the cervix and uterus respond to the dilatation of the cervix and the contraction of the uterus by altering the polarity of the afferent nerve fibres. This creates an action potential, in other words the 'sensation has been transferred into an electrical impulse' (Vander et al 1994: p 234). As a result of this information regarding these changes this makes the woman aware of pain sensation.

Action potential

The nerve cell is stimulated by the pain chemicals which alter the neurones' sodium and potassium channels by opening and closing them. In order for nerve transmission to occur depolarization and then repolarization take place in the nerve fibre. Sodium and potassium are positively charged, which means that there is a resultant exchange of positive charges into and out of the cell. Potassium ions inside the cell begin to exchange places with sodium. At a critical level the cell is depolarized – the inside of the cell becomes positive in relation to the outside of the cell. Repolarization takes place creating an equilibrium in the cell. This is reached when the sodium–potassium pump, as it is called, equalizes the potassium outside the cell membrane and the sodium inside the cell. The negative–positive balance returns to the neurone which is termed its resting potential. The depolarization and repolarization of the nerve fibre occur over a period of 0.5 m/s and facilitate the spread of information from one part of the nervous system to the next (Bullock 1992, Tortora & Grabowski 1992) (Fig. A.2). The nature of uterine contractions are such that they permit a certain amount of relaxation from pain for the woman when the uterus is relaxed. If contractions are frequent and strong the action potential of the nerve fibre builds up pain sensations increasing the pain intensity for the woman. Signals travel only in one direction, when the terminal of the nerve fibre is reached synapses occur where neurotransmitter substances facilitate nerve transmission across the gap in the nerve terminals. The nervous system thus forms a network of nerve fibres throughout the body, sending electrical impulses along the nerve fibres in order to transfer information along its system – like the wiring circuit in a house (Bloom & Lazerson 1988).

Nerve transmission

Nerve transmission is along fibres that conduct sensations in different strengths and at different speeds. These fibres are either A delta thinly myelinated fibres or C fibres which are unmyelinated fibres. It is the smaller C fibres, found in the deep viscera such as the uterus, which give rise to the deep prolonged pain of labour being stimulated by muscular contraction and chemical substances (Whipple 1990). Pain is transferred by action potentials along the nerve fibres to the dorsal horn of the spinal cord and thence to upward tracts to the central nervous system. As a result of the release of bradykinins and histamines and other pain-inducing substances at tissue level, substance P is also released. This is a neuropeptide and is released from the afferent nerves (Vander et al 1994) as part of the 'signalling process' of pain on its way to the dorsal horn of the spinal cord and could be termed a potentiator of pain sensation. As the action potential from the afferent neurones meets the spinal cord it enters by the posterior (dorsal) root and is transferred to the substantia gelatinosa at lamina or layers ii and iii of the grey matter of the spinal cord. These laminae decode various types of stimulus and transfer sensations to the higher centres of the brain via the anterior and lateral spinothalamic tracts which cross to the opposite side of the cord before ascending (Whipple 1990, Barasi 1991). Descending tracts from the brain returning to the spinal cord may make a modulating effect on the nerve transmission of pain. Naturally occurring endorphins at the spinal level act like exogenous opioids by modulating the pain response (Hung 1987, Barasi 1991) (Fig. A.3).

THE GATE THEORY OF PAIN

Pain modulation at the spinal cord is based on the fact that nerves may carry both excitatory information and inhibitory information. In competing at this level it modulates the sensation of the original pain stimulus at the substantia gelatinosa. Inhibition of pain at this level can occur naturally by the production of endorphins or by transcutaneous electrical nerve stimulation (Thibodeau 1990). Areas within the brain and substantia gelatinosa of the spinal cord have been identified and have been found to produce natural endorphins, morphine-like substances that bind to receptors in these areas to modulate pain sensation. β-endorphin is produced in the hypothalamic pituitary region of the brain and has been found to be increased in plasma and cerebrospinal fluid in pregnancy and parturition (Barasi 1991, Jacques 1994). These naturally occurring pain-modulating substances are an important source of pain relief for women in labour and may be stimulated by massage and TENS.

The process of pain initiation is summarized in Box 3.1.

PAIN AND HOMEOSTASIS

Any attempt to describe pain is complex, as each individual experiencing it will use different mechanisms and words to describe their feelings of pain. Keele et al (1983) describe it as 'an unpleasant sensory experience distinct from any other sensory modalities such as touch, warmth or cold' (p 394). It

---

Box 3.1 Summary of the process of pain initiation

◆ Chemicals or pressure stimulate the nerve endings
◆ An action potential is formed in the nerves
◆ The impulse travels along the nerves to the spinal cord and then to the central nervous system

may be described in the affective or psychological domain or the sensory domain. Ligaments are stretched and affected by levels of relaxin produced in pregnancy (Johnson & Everitt 1993), the growth of the uterus alters positions of internal organs and body stance is altered to accommodate the heavy uterus. In order for the body to maintain homeostasis when pain is experienced, the adrenal cortex responds to more adrenocorticotrophic hormone (ACTH). The release of cortisol stimulates the release of adrenaline and noradrenaline from the adrenal medulla, activating a rise in the pulse and respiratory rate. This has the effect of increasing oxygen levels to the tissues and maintaining cellular balance within the body (Bonica & Chadwick 1990, Thibodeau 1990) (Fig. A.4). Cortisol is increased as a response to the stress that is caused by the experience of pain, this may increase the length of the first stage of labour (Burns 1976). It also has a beneficial effect in that rises in cortisol increase the natural secretion of β-endorphins (Hung 1987). Although a rise of adrenaline and noradrenaline may have a beneficial effect on increasing pulse and respiratory rates, researchers have found that high levels may cause a delay in labour by diminishing uterine activity (Lederman et al 1978). These substances are also a reaction to developing stress as well as the physiological action within the body to pain.

FETAL–MATERNAL INTERACTIONS

The fetus, as it is dependent on the mother via the placenta, will also react to maternal circulatory changes, and a healthy full-term infant will respond to changes in its environment particularly in labour as uterine activity increases. A healthy infant will be able to balance these changes and maintain its homeostasis, but any deficit in the fetus will consequently affect its ability to maintain these homeostatic balances. The woman in labour requires adequate sources of glucose and energy. She needs to maintain an optimum circulation to support both herself and the fetus during the hours of labour. The rise in cortisol levels aids this. If the mother suffers vena-caval compression from lying in the dorsal position for vaginal examination or monitoring, or hypotension from the induction of an epidural the fetus may become compromised. This may cause a fetal hypoxia and acidosis as a result of an imbalance in the mother or poor uterine blood flow to the placenta. In the process of labour the mother may alter her respiratory rate in an attempt to cope with pain, in turn this will alter her respiratory gas balances and have its effect on the fetus by altering the rate of the exchange of gases available to the placenta (Bonica & Chadwick 1990). There seems to be some benefit to both mother and fetus in the use of effective pain relief in circumstances where the mother is extremely stressed.

PAIN DESCRIPTORS AND RESEARCH DESIGN

In order that pain may be analysed, pain descriptor charts have been devised and women have participated in research to clarify their experience of labour pain. Much of this research in recent years has been in the experience of pain, in order to develop a better understanding of it. These charts are detailed and require time to complete; various researchers have modified the questionnaires so that they are more suitable for women in labour. Much of the research has been performed retrospectively, with the possible disadvantage that memory and time alter true pain recall. The following are some of the statements used by 100 women in a large teaching hospital to identify the type of pain that they experienced in the first stage of labour. Women used varying adjectives in discussing the pain they experienced in labour: 'a dull ache in my lower back, stabbing pains, stabs of sharp pain down my thighs, it felt like I had eaten something bad'. Some women, although in the minority, stated that it was 'like bad wind' and 'not painful' (Bradford & Chamberlain 1995: p 36).

The McGill–Melzack pain questionnaire devised in 1975 measures the quality of pain under specific headings, sensory, affective and evaluative. The present pain intensity (PPI) measures the intensity of pain experienced by a scoring system between 0 and 5. The questionnaire was administered to people with specific pain syndromes, two of which were labour pain and menstrual pain. Menstrual pain was described as cramping and aching while labour pain was pounding, shooting, stabbing, sharp, cramping and aching. The affective component of pain was described as tiring and sickening for menstrual pain and tiring, exhausting and fearful for labour pain. It is interesting to note that the word fear is used in labour to describe the pain experienced, this justifies the definition of the pain experience as being influenced by psychological factors and also highlights all the research recently into support in labour and its benefits to women in labour (Hodnett 1997). In comparing the intensity of labour pain to other pain experienced, labour pain was said on the rating scale to be worse than cancer pain and phantom limb pain (Melzack & Wall 1991).

Other methods of pain evaluation used Likert-type scales or visual analogue scales such as Huskinsson (1983) describes. A vertical or horizontal line 10 cm in length is represented on paper with end points suggesting 'no pain' and 'severe pain' and the appropriate mark is put in a position as to the severity of the pain experienced by the person. This is then measured by the researcher and compared to other scores. This tool has been proven to be an accurate method of measuring pain over various time scales (Huskinsson 1983). It is quick and easy to administer in the labour room and because of its simplicity does not take much thought or consideration on the recipient's part to complete.

Bonnel & Boureau (1985) researched pain in labour by using a pain rating index as described above and a behavioural index (Present Behavioural Intensity, PBI). One hundred primigravidae were observed in labour where the observer noted the way that pain was expressed at various cervical dilatations and rated this on a scale of 1–4. Following labour, self-report measures were taken on a three-point scale 'agreeable, bearable or unbearable'. Pain intensity was also assessed by the woman and her midwife, as 'no pain, moderate pain, severe pain' following the birth. This brought validity to the PBI scales reported by the observer in labour.

In attempting to research the quality and experience of pain in labour it must be approached in such a way that all factors are taken into consideration. Pain is a multidimensional experience and therefore needs to be approached by the researchers in a multidimensional way. Most research design in pain in childbirth has used the sensory and affective dimensions of pain against such variables as stage in labour, cervical dilatation, whether primigravida or multiparous, pain expectations, support in labour, length of labour, previous pain experience. Some have been descriptive studies analysing labour events against measurement of pain. Lowe (1991) used five psychological and seven physiological variables during early, active, transitional and the second stage of labour. Questionnaires were administered by a nurse research assistant in the labour room but some of this data was difficult for the participant to complete because of the speed of labour. Other data was acquired by interview. Pain-scoring charts were easily administered to the client except in transitional labour and during the birth. These scores are nearly always obtained early in the postnatal period and are more a memory of the pain of labour which could well be influenced at this time by the tiredness and memory of experiences of the birth process as a whole. Brown et al (1989) studied the characteristics of labour pain at various cervical dilatations using the McGill pain questionnaire, and found women were using similar descriptors to other researchers. During the first stage of labour primigravidae experienced higher pain scores than those of multigravidae (Brown et al 1989). This may be because better coping mechanisms had been developed with previous experience of pain in labour for the second-time mothers. In the research design it must be considered that the use of a research assistant will in some way impinge on the perception of the event by the mother and may introduce bias (Polit & Hungler 1993).

Qualitative data is an essential component of this type of research as it adds focus and develops theories, and is holistic. It is however subjective and leaves some individual interpretation for the researchers. The collection of quantitative data from the pain-rating scales tests theories, brings an element of control, is objective and concise (Burns & Grove 1987). A combination of the two research techniques gives a balance to the research of pain in labour.

CONCLUSION

This chapter has attempted to clarify the process of pain as applied to labour, what causes the pain, how it is transferred and how the body attempts to modify pain by explaining the gate theory of pain process. Pain research in midwifery centres around women's experiences. It is difficult to assess pain in a scientific way as women vary so much in their pain perception and so many factors impinge on the birth experience. It is very evident from the papers written in the last couple of years that support is all important in the labour process, in particular a trained support partner for the woman to enable her to feel confident in the environment in which she gives birth. It is important that midwives working within hospital environments make the experience of birth as pleasant as possible by being supportive and 'with the woman'. It should be a day for her to remember.

ANNOTATED BIBLIOGRAPHY

Chard T, Grudinskas JD (eds) 1994 The uterus. Cambridge University Press, Cambridge

A well written but complex book covering the anatomy and the physiology of the uterus to great depth.

Mander R 1998 Pain in childbearing and its control. Blackwell Scientific, Oxford

Written by a midwife, giving a broad view of pain in childbearing.

REFERENCES

Austin CR, Short RV 1990 Reproduction in mammals no 3. Hormonal control of reproduction 2nd edn. Cambridge University Press, Cambridge
Barasi S 1991 The physiology of pain. Surgical Nurse 4 (5): 14–20
Bernal A, Lopez 1996 Parturition. In: Hillier SG, Kitchener HC, Neilson JP (eds) Scientific essentials of reproductive medicine. WB Saunders, London, ch 3
Bhalla RC, Sandorn RM, Korenman SG 1972 Hormonal interactions in the uterus: inhibition of isoproterenol-induced accumulation of adenosine 3':5'-cyclic monophosphate by oxytocin and prostaglandins. Proceedings of the National Academy of Sciences USA 69: 3761–3764
Bloom FE, Lazerson A 1988 Brain mind and behaviour, 2nd edn. WH Freeman, New York
Bonica JF, Chadwick HS 1990 Labour pain. In: Wall PD, Melzack R (eds) Textbook of pain. Churchill Livingstone, London, ch 34
Bonnel AM, Boureau F 1985 Labour pain assessment: validity of a behavioural index. Pain 22, pp 81–90
Bradford N, Chamberlain G 1995 Pain relief in childbirth. Harper Collins, London
British National Formulary 1996 British Medical Association and Royal Pharmacological Society of Great Britain. The Pharmaceutical Press, London
Brown ST, Campbell D, Kurtz A 1989 Characteristics of labour pain at two stages of cervical dilatation. Pain 38: 289–295

Bullock BL 1992 Pain. In: Bullock BL, Rosendahl PP (eds) Pathophysiology adaptations and alterations in function, 3rd edn. Lippincott, Philadelphia, ch 51

Burns JK 1976 Relationship between blood cortisol levels and the duration of human labour. Journal of Physiology 254: 12

Burns N, Grove SK 1987 The practice of nursing research. WB Saunders, London

Carston ME 1973 Prostaglandins and cellular calcium transport in the human pregnant uterus. American Journal of Obstetrics and Gynaecology 117: 824–832

Dick Read G 1950 Childbirth without fear. William Heinemann, London

Egater CH, Husslein P 1992 Biochemistry of myometrial contractility. Baillière's clinical obstetrics and gynaecology 6: 755–768

Fuèntes A, Spaziani EP, O'Brien WF 1996 The expression of cyclooxygenase-2 (COX-2) in amnion and decidua following spontaneous labour. Prostaglandins 52: 361–367

Gibb DMF 1993 Measurement of uterine activity in labour. British Journal of Obstetrics and Gynaecology, 100 (suppl 9): 28–31

Goff KJ 1993 Initiation of parturition. American Journal of Maternal and Child Nursing 18 (suppl): 23–30 Sept/Oct, pp 7–13

Hodnett ED 1997 Support from caregivers during childbirth. In: Neilson JP, Crowther CA, Hodnett ED, Hofmeyr GJ, Keirse MJNC (eds). Pregnancy and childbirth module of the Cochrane Database of Systematic Reviews. The Cochrane Collaboration, Oxford

Hung TT 1987 The role of endogenous opioids in pregnancy and analgesia. Seminars in Reproductive Endocrinology May: 161–168

Huskinsson EC 1983 Visual Analogue Scales. In: Melzack R (ed) Pain measurement and assessment. Raven, New York, p 33

Huszar G, Roberts JM 1982 Biochemistry and pharmacology of the myometrium and labour: regulation at the cellular and molecular levels. American Journal of Obstetrics and Gynaecology 142: 225–235

Jacques A 1994 Physiology of pain. British Journal of Nursing 3: 607–610

Javert CT, Hardy JD 1950 Measurement of pain intensity in labour and its physiologic, neurologic and pharmacologic implications. American Journal of Obstetrics and Gynecology 60: 552–563

Johnson M, Everitt B 1993 Essential reproduction, 3rd edn. Blackwell Scientific, London

Keele CA, Neil E, Joels N 1983 Samson Wright's applied physiology, 13th edn. Oxford University Press, Oxford

Kirkham M 1991 Antenatal learning. Nursing Times, 87 (9): 67

Lederman RP, Lederman E, Work B, McCann D 1978 The relationship of maternal anxiety, plasma catecholamines, and plasma cortisol to progression in labour. American Journal of Gynaecology 1: 495–500

Lowe NK 1991 Critical predictors of sensory and affective pain during four phases of labour. Journal of Psychosomatic Obstetrics and Gynaecology 12: 193–208

Llewellyn-Jones D 1990 Fundamentals in obstetrics and gynaecology, 5th edn. Faber and Faber, London

Mitchell MD, Flint APF, Bibby J et al 1977 Rapid increases in plasma prostaglandin concentration after vaginal examination and amniotomy. British Medical Journal 2: 1183

Melzack R, Wall P 1991 The challenge of pain. Penguin Books, Harmondsworth, Middlesex, p 41

McCaffery M 1983 Nursing the patient in pain. Harper and Row, London

Moir C 1939 The nature of the pain of labour. Journal of Obstetrics and Gynaecology of the British Empire 46: 409–424

Niven C, Gijspers K 1984 A study of labour pain using the McGill pain questionnaire. Social Science and Medicine 19: 1347–1351

Polit DE, Hungler BP 1993 Essentials of nursing research, 3rd edn. JB Lippincott, Philadelphia

Ramsey E 1994 Anatomy of the uterus. In: Chard T, Grundzinskas JD (eds) The uterus. Cambridge University Press, Cambridge, ch 2

Raphael-Leff J 1991 Psychological processes of childbearing. Chapman & Hall, London

Robinson JS, Challis JRG, Thorburn GD 1977 Initiation of labour. In: Chamberlain G (ed) Contemporary obstetrics and gynaecology. Northwood Publications, pp 157–163

Steer PJ 1991 The genital system. In: Hytten F, Chamberlain G (eds) Clinical physiology in obstetrics, 2nd edn. Blackwell Scientific, Oxford, ch 12

Stjernquist M, Sjöberg NO 1994 Neurotransmitters in the myometrium. In: Chard T, Grundzinskas JD (eds) The uterus. Cambridge University Press, Cambridge, ch 9

Thibodeau GA 1990 Antony's textbook of anatomy and physiology, 13th edn. Times Mirror/Mosby College Publishing, St Louis

Tortora GJ, Grabowski SR 1992 Principles of anatomy and physiology, 7th edn. Harper Collins, College Publications, New York
Vander AJ, Sherman JH, Luciano DS 1994 Human physiology, 6th edn. McGraw-Hill, New York
Whipple B 1990 Neurophysiology of pain. Orthopaedic Nursing 9(4): 21–25
Williams PL, Warwick R, Dyson M, Bannister LH (eds) 1989 Gray's anatomy, 37th edn. Churchill Livingstone, Edinburgh

4

Psychology of pain in normal labour

Helen Crafter

INTRODUCTION

It quickly becomes apparent to student midwives and other health professionals entering clinical practice that pain is not the same experience for everyone. Some women will sail through their labour, perhaps not even recognizing labour pain as such, while others will request epidural anaesthesia with early contractions. This chapter will address the purpose of labour pain and explore why the experience of pain is so variable by looking at psychological and cultural differences through which pain sensation is

43

perceived and interpreted. Finally evidence of women's experiences of labour will be gathered from the literature and explored for common themes as to what the major influences on pain perception and sensation are, and whether such influences can (and should) be manipulated by women and birth attendant to enhance women's experiences of labour.

A positivist framework to labour pain and discomfort is adopted. This means that the chapter will seek to examine the benefits rather than a more medical approach of viewing pain in normal physiological labour as a problem which requires control and obliteration. Labour pain is however acknowledged as, by many women's testimony, one of the most painful experiences that a human is called upon to endure.

WHAT IS NORMAL LABOUR?

Normal labour is a difficult concept to define. Such a definition should obviously include the process of uterine contractions which dilate the cervix, and the descent and birth of a fetus undamaged by the birth process. However placing a strict timescale on normality has great limitations and can be inaccurate if a labour although long by medical definition, poses no risk or damage to the mother or fetus. Yet if the definition includes a timescale psychologically acceptable to the mother, is a labour that becomes unbearable after 6 hours abnormal? Almost all health professionals would argue not. A further problem in defining normality is that if a timescale is not absolute and labour is allowed to continue in the absence of abnormal observations, damage may not be obvious until the labour is completed. Yet a labour is surely not 'normal' if it leaves a woman so physically and emotionally drained that she cannot care adequately for her newborn infant or even enjoy her baby's first few hours of life. Almost all textbooks will therefore state a maximum time within which 'normal' labour is said to occur to avoid the complications of maternal and fetal exhaustion; one of the shortest is O'Driscoll & Meagher's (1993) timescale (12 hours from time of delivery suite admission to completion of the second stage) to that of Morrin (1997), who gives a maximum length of normal labour as 24 hours. However, such general criteria do not attempt to take into account women's individual wishes and experiences and, for many health professionals, will therefore represent guidelines for discussion with the women in their care rather than absolute rules.

WHAT IS THE PURPOSE OF LABOUR PAIN?

Types and purposes of pain in a variety of human conditions are well documented in the literature, one of the most notable and frequently referenced being Melzack & Wall's *The Challenge of Pain* (1988). However the experience of pain during the normal and natural process of birth is unique (in that normally pain is a warning sign of tissue damage) and therefore it is useful to explore why labouring women feel pain and what its purpose is. Many people have deliberated on these questions and made suggestions, ranging from 'Eve's Curse', which suggests women are punished for Eve's sin of tempting Adam out of the Garden of Eden, to the idea that pain is only perceived by women who expect it (or have over-high expectations of being able to overcome it), are over-anxious or are not performing breathing exercises correctly.

Let's turn this around; what would happen if labour produced no pain or discomfort? Consider reflective scenario 4.1. This scenario is intended to illustrate the positive benefit of discomfort in labour, which would have warned Anna that birth was imminent and given her time to prepare herself physically and psychologically for it. It would have allowed her to 'nest' by going to a more private place with her helpers, it would have allowed her to concentrate on the task in hand (getting the baby born) and it perhaps would have enabled her and her helpers to recognize a deviation from normal such as a dangerously prolonged labour or the continuous pain present during placental abruption, had these occurred. Would any sensation other than pain persuade the vast majority of women to stop what they were doing, however important it felt, and prepare mentally and physically for the imminent birth?

Perhaps our next question should be that if pain can be perceived as a fundamentally positive aspect of physiologically normal labour, why do so many women find it unmanageable and seek recourse to drugs, and why do

---

Reflective scenario 4.1

Anna, 37 weeks pregnant, wants to work as late as possible into her pregnancy to accumulate paid time off after the birth with her baby. She is having a particularly busy day spending much of it on her feet, as a couple of her colleagues are off sick. As she knows it is normal for the baby's head to engage in the pelvis at around this time the heaviness she feels in her groin only serves to excite her – surely a sign of normality and a response to so much physical activity.

She is really looking forward to her best friend Jay's hen night this evening, straight after work. Later, as she dances the night away, despite a feeling of increasing tiredness, she feels an urgent need to visit the toilet. However half way across the crowded dance floor she just manages to catch her baby as he makes his slippery entrance into the world...

a few find it so severe that the memory of the experience gives them long-term psychological problems? To look for answers to these questions it is useful to look at older societies where birth has been untouched by modern medicine and women receive social support, massage and other non-pharmacological methods of pain relief in the absence of drugs (for instance those described by Goldsmith 1990). The women Goldsmith describes often have quite different perceptions of labour pain and discomfort to western women, sometimes having no concept of pain as such, although all recognize the need to find a suitable environment in which to give birth. Although it is easy to romanticize the latter as 'more natural' and superior this is perhaps an unfair comparison; the pain that most women describe during their labour is very real and in cultures where pain is not generally tolerated stoically it is not helpful, nor accurate, to shrug it off as 'all in the mind', or a result of not preparing properly for the birth experience. However it can be demonstrated through anthropological studies that *attitudes* to pain are crucial to the way in which it is perceived. Could it be that the *nature of society* and a woman's *cultural heritage* imprint on her a 'normal' response to pain, and that responses will differ for women living in different parts of the world, or from different cultural backgrounds? Furthermore, do the attitudes health professionals bring to the birthing room, and their own culturally based beliefs influence the experiences individual women undergo? The historical and contemporary literature from the fields of anthropology and psychology would suggest that this is so, and that attitudes are far more influential than many health professionals appreciate.

The considerations of attitude and cultural heritage are demonstrated in a study by Wetering & Eskes (1988), who compared the expectations of American and Dutch women to pain in their forthcoming labours. They found that 54% of the Americans expected labour to be very painful compared to 29% of the Dutch women in the sample, and 62% of the American women expected to receive pain-relieving drugs compared to 20% of Dutch women. When the researchers returned shortly after the births they found that 62% of the Dutch women had received no medication in labour but only 16% of the American mothers had managed without. They concluded that the expectation of pain in labour was to some extent a self-fulfilling prophesy, and cultural attitudes towards birth may dictate women's expectations to some extent. The researchers comment that in the USA birth is seen as a medical event whereas in the Netherlands it is seen more as a social event, home birth being a common occurrence (although the women in this study gave birth in hospital).

In summary, labour pain appears to have a very necessary purpose; yet the interpretation of the sensations that women experience are open to different, and very wide perceptions.

THE HISTORY OF OUR UNDERSTANDING OF THE PSYCHOLOGICAL ASPECTS OF PAIN

That pain has a psychological dimension as well as a physical one is a relatively new concept which only really started to gain acceptance in the western world this century (Ogden 1996). The disassociation of pain from the psyche was indeed strengthened in the late nineteenth and early twentieth centuries when the use of chemical analgesics for severe, often intractable pain became more widespread. This made the acknowledgement of 'physical' pain and its relief for sufferers much more positive to health professionals in their wish to cure it than the more variable and less easy to quantify psychological aspects involved in the perception of pain.

The concept of pain as a purely physical experience had also been encouraged by such early theorists as Descartes in the seventeenth century. His comparatively simple idea was that a pain stimulus would produce a response, the link between the cause of pain and the brain being automatic (Ogden 1996). This physical concept of pain was developed by Muller in 1842 and Von Frey in 1894–95 (Melzack & Wall 1988), further discouraging people to consider whether pain was a far more complicated process.

Although the psychological aspects of pain had come to be acknowledged early in the twentieth century in some quarters, one of the first widely accepted theories to encapsulate this idea came from Melzack & Wall in 1965 (Melzack & Wall 1988) in their gate control theory. The previous biomedical models of pain were adapted to include expectations, experience, mood and behaviour, which placed pain as a perception and experience in itself rather than a physical sensation. The 'gate', which is said to exist at the spinal cord level, opens to raise the perception of pain or closes to decrease it under the influence of physical, emotional and behavioural factors. For example, major injury, anxiety and boredom may increase pain and a requirement for analgesia, whereas a state of relaxation and distraction will alleviate pain. This theory has gained popular widespread support, not least from those seeking to understand labour discomfort and pain. It is of interest to note that it has received little critique in the literature and has yet to be effectively challenged by an alternative model which attains similar universal agreement.

THE HISTORY AND 'HERSTORY' OF PSYCHOLOGICAL ASPECTS OF PAIN IN LABOUR

Until the advent of modern medicine and its ability to relieve pain pharmacologically, it probably never occurred to most women that labour was anything other than something they were required to experience in order to produce children. Indeed, many were probably so afraid of losing their own life, or that of the baby, that pain may have been perceived as a side issue rather than an important issue in itself. However, women have campaigned alongside doctors throughout history to find safe analgesic drugs (Carter & Duriez 1986), and once drugs are made available to women to control pain, it is a common observation that many women in physiologically normal labour choose to have them even when they are aware of the dangers and disadvantages. This must be seen as testimony to the severe nature of pain that labouring women feel in the western world, particularly (but not exclusively) during a long labour or one in which the fetus occupies a suboptimal position. However it is also likely that the belief and overwhelming trust that women from such societies have placed in clinical medicine in the last hundred years or so underlie their acceptance of a model that seeks to obliterate, or at least control, pain and discomfort rather than approach it as a catalyst to develop the power to overcome a challenge, and be strengthened by it.

In the mid-nineteenth century ether and chloroform became available for labouring women, the first drugs felt to be safe enough for both the mother and fetus. However, because women did not practise medicine at this time and midwives were not acknowledged as professionals, they had little say as to how 'safe' a drug should be. It is now known that many women in normal labour died as a result of respiratory depression brought on by the administration of these gases (Carter & Duriez 1986). Because they had to be administered by a doctor, who had to be paid privately, ether and chloroform were on the whole available only to wealthy women. Poorer women continued to depend on a 'handy woman' or uncertified midwife who had learned her trade from observation, experience and having her own babies. Alternatively (or perhaps in addition) she may have had female relatives in attendance. The comfort this social support provided for many women may be broadly recognized as instinctive knowledge by women that physical comfort and emotional support go an enormous way in providing for psychological needs in labour, and impact on perception of pain. Women of the time will not have had the means or ability to read about the advantages of such companionship, but its existence in society demonstrates implicit knowledge.

In the 1930s a doctor, Grantly Dick Read, had begun to question the practice of administering strong analgesia and anaesthesia to labouring women. By this time the dangers of chloroform were acknowledged and 'Twilight Sleep', a mixture of injectable scopolamine and morphine, had been developed. However the effect of this cocktail of drugs could not be predicted for individual women and Dick Read was one of a number of outspoken critics. While others continued the search for drugs with fewer side-effects, Dick Read proposed that the pain could be adequately controlled using psychoprophylaxis – a 'mind over matter' attitude where if women were relieved of fear and tension, their pain would diminish to a level they could cope with, or disappear.

Dick Read cites a single experience that altered his previously medically orthodox approach to labour pain. While attending a woman in a poverty-stricken area of London, he offered her chloroform as the baby's head appeared. The woman kindly and firmly declined the offer. When he asked her after the birth why she would not take the mask, the woman thought for a moment, looked at the 'old woman' who had been attending her, and replied, 'It didn't hurt. It wasn't meant to, was it doctor?' Dick Read went on to observe many physiologically normal labours, some in which the woman appeared free of pain and some in which the woman experienced unbearable pain. It was his observation that fear was the underlying factor that led to the perception of severe pain; that fear of anticipation of problems and fear of the pain itself initiated the mechanism of protective action by the body and this included muscle tension. He proposed that such tension closes the uterus and cervix and increases resistance to dilatation, whereas in the normal state the muscles are relaxed and free of tension. This resistance leads to pain because the nerves to the uterus respond to excessive tension (Dick Read 1943). Dick Read also records his observations of women who overcome the fear–tension–pain cycle through antental education as being uplifted and exalted by labour, rather than dragged down and overcome by its intensity.

However it was only a matter of time before practically all women were given the option of pharmacological pain relief in labour. The inception of the National Health Service in the UK in 1948, and generally available private health schemes in the rest of the western world, have been partially responsible for the demise of the autonomous midwife who had the competence and confidence to 'get women through labour', and the growth of the medicalization of birth with its power to control and sanitize birth into a pain-free experience of short duration.

The medicalization of birth, which has grown quickly as analgesia for parturient women has become more widely available (making possible otherwise painful and difficult procedures such as routine amniotomy and instrumental delivery) began the trend to view birth as a medical rather than a social event. As a consequence, psychosocial aspects of the birth experience have received less attention and the control of pain and labour have become the focus of intrapartum care. The trend of medicalization reached its peak in the 1960s and 1970s in the west when birth had almost completely moved into the hospital, women were often delivered by a midwife or doctor they hardly knew (and certainly not personally) and all family members were excluded from the birth room. Not surprisingly against this background, epidural analgesia has steadily grown in popularity since its general introduction in the British delivery suite in the late 1960s (Bevis 1984), and the race continues to this day to find effective analgesia which is free from side-effects. However, debate also continues in the media about whether pain relief presently available, with its many undesirable side-effects, should be encouraged or even readily available for women in normal labour, or whether women would be generally better served by a culture of good education and support which enables them to approach labour as a positive experience through which the majority can personally triumph.

Different writers have developed different approaches as to how the psychology of labour pain can be explored. One such writer is Adrienne Rich who asked in her feminist critique *Of Woman Born* if physical pain can be distinguished from fear, and suggests that the answer will be different depending on the cultural group one studies (Rich 1986). It may be true in western society that fear of pain and discomfort in labour is so ingrained that it becomes impossible to move wholesale into a more accepting understanding of pain, although individuals will no doubt always exist in all societies who feel minimal discomfort, and others will successfully train themselves to bear labour without drugs. Rich also discusses the distinction between the pain of suffering, characterized by pain yet leading to growth and enlightenment, and affliction, where pain can be endless and with no apparent purpose. She draws on history to reveal a picture of the afflictions endured by women; first having no means to prevent conception, and the cycle of unceasing birth year after year, and then the later prison of unconsciousness, numbed sensations, amnesia and complete passivity in the birth process. She argues that pain as a label has been applied indiscriminately to the range of sensations that women have during the birth process, thereby denying the complexity of the individual woman's experience (Rich 1986). However, while not providing answers to the dilemmas posed by modern medicine of the travails of the labouring woman, neither does Rich see 'non-literate' societies as having superior attitudes to pregnancy and birth.

WOMEN'S EXPERIENCES OF LABOUR PAIN

Women experience the complexities of labour in numerous ways. Most will describe it as painful, but will describe the pain in different ways. For instance in a Swedish study of 278 women 41% described it as the 'worst imaginable' pain, but 28% experienced the pain in a positive way (Scopesi et al 1997). Kitzinger (1997) points out that in studies the amount of pain a woman endures bears little relation to the satisfaction she feels. Some women report a great deal of pain, but have a positive experience of birth, while others report little pain, but have a negative birth experience. Kitzinger concludes that exclusively focusing on the issue of pain in labour does not record with accuracy women's experiences of labour.

Ranta et al (1996) looked at the pain experiences of grande multiparae (women who had at least five previous deliveries) and found that they described less pain than primigravidae with similar cervical dilatation in early labour but intense pain during the birth which was much greater than that reported by the primigravidae in the study (40% of whom had epidural anaesthesia). However, none of the grande multigravidae received epidurals and 47% of them regarded their analgesia as insufficient.

An article which perhaps gives the most vivid description of women's experiences of labour, of descriptive research so favoured by Kitzinger, is that of Halldorsdottir & Karlsdottir (1996) set in Iceland. A sample of 14 mothers with healthy babies were asked for their perspective of birth. The researchers' focus concentrated on the experience of labour and birth rather than that of pain and it is interesting to note how few of the women's comments relate to pain, considering the attention it is given in professional journals generally.

INFLUENCES ON THE PERCEPTION OF LABOUR PAIN

The role of culture

Although cultural issues are addressed in Chapter 5, it is worth considering the relationship between culture and its psychological interpretation. Culture is seen by social anthropologists as the fabric of beliefs of a society involving religious beliefs, myths, art, manners, dress, etc. which holds that society together and is transmitted through the generations in spoken and unspoken ways. Culture serves to enable people to belong to a group; the self esteem of the individual and the group is enhanced through a sense of belonging and being accepted as one of the group. Culture teaches us how to perceive and interpret the world around us, within a specific set of shared meanings. Conformity has a strong attraction to most individuals as it enables us to reap the benefits of the cultural group or groups we most identify with.

Labour pain may therefore be viewed through a cultural perspective, although the interpretation of cultural norms always involves subjective explanation and elucidation.

In the labour and birth setting, part of the culture is expressed through the environment and how this is organized. In the UK, for instance, 98% of women give birth in hospital (Office for National Statistics 1997). Individual purpose-built rooms are usually set aside and furnished. The furnishings give important clues as to the culture, or social meaning the setting portrays. Some hospitals provide home-like furniture and decorations – double bed, pine cupboards, pastel wallpaper and no or little evidence of technological aids (fetal monitors, resuscitaires, delivery trolleys, etc), which are accessed only when required.

Yet each furnishing which would not be found in the home indicates a cultural shift from the social birth environment. A single bed indicates that the woman's labour partner is not welcome to rest comfortably with her. An obstetric bed indicates that the environment seeks to ensure the comfort of the health professional in delivering the baby, rather than that of the woman. A bed in the middle of the room as a dominant feature of the birth environment suggests that it is expected to be used by the labouring woman, whereas a bed at the side of the room, or alternative furniture such as a birthing stool, rocking chair, bean bag and mats, indicate that the woman is not necessarily expected to labour in any one place. (Beds often take central position in a bedroom at home because they are the central feature; bedrooms are primarily for sleeping in.)

Furnishings in a hospital delivery room give women subliminal messages about how the presiding culture expects them to behave. As we expect to share cultural meanings and culture seeks to make us feel an important part of a group, there is a strong need for the woman to behave as she feels her supporters expect of her. Cardiotocograph machines, epidural trolleys, spotlights attached to the ceiling and 'anaesthetic room paint' (traditionally green) will all serve to give women a cultural picture of behaviour expectation. For a woman in a room with medicalized surroundings who desires a drug-free labour and birth, the experience of not conforming to an established and very visual pattern may well increase her levels of stress and this in turn may lower her threshold for tolerating pain.

What do mothers teach us?

Although impossible to prove, it seems likely that girls and women subconsciously absorb many of their own mothers' and female relatives' attitudes about labour and birth. If a young girl grows up in an environment where childbirth is feared or not spoken about she may be exposed to feelings that encourage fear in her own beliefs. Conversely, if she grows up in an environment where childbirth and its process are seen as positive events, her mother's experiences are freely discussed and birth pain is not generally feared, she is much more likely to approach all the sensations of birth more confidently and positively. However sisters can behave very differently in labour, and such an influence on women's attitudes must surely be tenuous and very complicated.

The role of psychological preparation for birth in reducing the physical experience of pain and the need for pain-relieving drugs

In 1981 Melzack et al demonstrated in their small study that prepared childbirth training (PCT) designed to reduce fear, anxiety and tension did decrease the pain that women felt in labour, and that women who had had education were less likely to require pain relief than those who did not. The classes consisted of instruction in physiology, breathing exercises and relaxation techniques. The researchers also found a difference in women's pain rating in labour depending on who their instructor was, and further questioning of the woman suggested that this was positively related to the enthusiasm of their teacher. However these findings have been partly refuted by Simkin (1995) in her review of published trials. She suggests that there is no evidence that attendance at antenatal classes is linked with a reduction in pain, but there is some evidence that attendance is associated with a reduction in the use of pain medication.

Hillan (1992) in a small study of women's views of caesarean section found that 50% of respondents criticized antenatal classes. They felt that the teaching in their classes had not prepared them for the experience of labour. Many had expected to use breathing techniques and labour positions taught in the classroom but were shocked at the intensity of their contractions, for which they did not feel prepared. Set beside Melzack's study, it may be seen that the quality of antenatal education is crucial to the way women perceive pain. If they believe the purpose of breathing exercises is to make the pain go away or be diminished, they may feel very misled and the subsequent lack of control they feel at being overcome by the pain experience may actually increase their physical experience of pain.

Therefore preparing women for the intensity of contractions, without inducing fear (and preferably reducing it), alongside teaching and practising coping mechanisms may be the key to effective antenatal education which aims to reduce the amount of pain relief required by women who would prefer to manage without.

Type of labour

The difficulty of defining normal labour has already been discussed. For some women the length of active labour will not be important as long as they feel able to cope, while for others a relatively short labour will feel unmanageable, particularly if it is characterized by acute sleep deprivation or persistent backache.

The nature of support in labour

Support in labour by health professionals can take many forms. However the requirements of labouring women from their carers should be the most important consideration in defining the nature of such support. Hutton (1994) reporting on a series of discussion groups with recent users of the maternity services in the UK found support to be giving explanations, encouragement and progress reports, giving undivided attention and consulting women about their wishes. Women also mentioned being listened to and taken seriously, having their right to choose respected and health professionals who have a belief that women have the ability to give birth without intervention.

The evidence suggests that support from a midwife whom the woman has got to know and trust during her pregnancy leads to a lower requirement for pain-relieving medication (for instance Rowley et al 1995, McCourt & Page 1996). However evidence also exists which suggests that it does not necessarily have to be a health professional providing support to make labour psychologically more manageable. A meta-analysis of randomized controlled trials by Klaus & Kennell (1997) into the effect on women of the continuous presence of a trained support person who had no previous social bond with the woman (known as a doula) demonstrated a lower requirement for medications for pain relief. A possible conclusion of Klaus & Kennell's work is that such emotional support and physical comfort measures enable women to cope better with labour pain by reducing fear and anxiety.

Klaus & Kennell in this study also compared the support that the baby's father offered to that of the doula. They found that doulas on the whole remained physically closer to women than the father and talked and touched women more. However when a doula accompanied a couple the father offered greater support to his partner. Although the presence of the father is acknowledged by Klaus & Kennell as an important emotional factor in labour, it is the presence of a doula which confers the greater benefits on outcome measures, with reduction in the use of pain relief being just one.

Place of birth and its effect on the experience of pain

It is difficult to find credible work which states whether or not pain feels strong and unmanageable, or bearable and manageable depending on place of birth. Studies do tell us that women labouring at home use less pharmacological pain relief (for instance Chamberlain et al 1997) but tend not to go so far as to attempt to demonstrate that women at home are in less pain than those labouring in hospital. Indeed pain is all perception; there is no objective test for others to accurately measure an individual's level of pain and, given previous studies discussed in this chapter, a reduced requirement for analgesia does not equate to women describing the pain as less; rather it becomes more manageable. Some studies seek to apply physical tests such as blood endorphin levels when assessing labour pain, but because of the complicated array of hormones present during labour biophysicists have yet to understand their complex relationship, let alone how a woman's psyche affects her endocrine interactions (Jowitt 1993).

Studies which look at women's experience of pain generally demonstrate that women at home are more likely to feel relaxed and in control (Davies et al 1996, Chamberlain et al 1997), experience less intervention, particularly induction and augmentation, and use less pharmacological analgesia (Chamberlain et al 1997). Inevitably these factors play into each other and affect the way women perceive pain.

Attitudes of health professionals to labour pain

It is well referenced that the attitudes and behaviour of health professionals attending and supporting women during pregnancy and labour will influence the way in which each woman perceives her labour and the choices she makes (or feels unable to make) as to how her labour proceeds in terms of the positions she adopts, the coping mechanisms she uses and the support she requests from her helpers.

The testimony of Susan (Halldorsdottir & Karlsdottir 1996) and her experience of a 'woman centred' midwife demonstrates vividly how sensitive health professionals can transform the experience of a woman in labour from that of a passive recipient into an active participant:

> *Then suddenly this midwife [came], and somehow she helped me to work with … you know to be on top of the wave instead of being in the middle of a huge surge. It was as if I was suddenly on a surfboard on top of the wave. All of a sudden I just stood there and I could feel that I was in control, I managed to work with my body, instead of feeling overpowered by something I couldn't handle. It was truly amazing to see the difference in having a midwife who was task-orientated, who was mainly concerned with the pains and then to have a midwife who was woman-orientated. Her attention was first and foremost on me … It was as if she positioned herself by my side and tried to figure out how I perceived things. (Susan, 40, mother of two)*

The ability to exude subtle confidence in a woman's ability to overcome her pain is a talent many midwives and doctors develop with experience, yet this ability is dependent on the health professional's underlying positive attitude towards the purpose of the pain itself within a holistic understanding of the process of labour.

However there is also a need to acknowledge that some women remain fearful of labour pain at its onset. The approach of health professionals in this situation further influences such women's pain perception. Green et al (1998) in a sample of 825 women who gave birth in the South East of England in April and May 1987 found that 16% of multigravidae questioned before delivery thought that a drug-free labour would be unbearably painful, compared to 7% of primigravidae. A previous experience of labour does not always reduce fear and in some cases it may exaggerate it. Women are known to highly value health professionals taking their views and beliefs seriously (Hutton 1994).

In a large study of perceptions of pain and pain relief in women and their professional attendants, Rajan (1993) demonstrated that the level of agreement about effectiveness was quite low. She suggests that midwives may tend to minimize the suffering women undergo to make life more comfortable for themselves, and this in itself causes problems for labouring women in that they can feel misunderstood.

Professional maternity care has its own cultural values and is at present in a state of cultural change. On the one hand the Department of Health's 'Changing Childbirth Report' (1993) encourages health professionals to make each woman the focus of maternity care, encouraging her to feel that she is in control of what is happening to her and able to make decisions about her care. Yet in practice many midwives and doctors, especially those who are hospital based, feel the weight of medical doctrine, impelled or instructed to use technology sometimes at odds with research based evidence and practice or the needs and wishes of a particular woman. Such divergent ideas and practices in intrapartum care inevitably affect the attitudes developed in health professionals, particularly those in the early stages of their career.

Public awareness of labour and birth issues

The 9 months of pregnancy seem a very short time for a woman and her partner to consider the many issues around birth and parenting before these events actually happen. For a woman who has given very little thought to labour and birth before getting pregnant, there is an enormous amount of information and self exploration to be done if she has the desire to. It can be impossible to make decisions without information and understanding on which to base them, and lack of information may also lead to increased fear about the process of labour, resulting in an enhanced perception of pain.

Increasing public awareness about birth issues, especially in the population's potential parents, can only serve to enlighten people and help them to understand some of the issues involved. The longer young people have to digest and explore knowledge, the better informed and able to develop their knowledge and understanding they will be when they come to have children themselves.

The media perform a vital function in exploring issues of public interest and it is important that midwives as well as other health professionals exploit this communication system in order to discuss and constantly challenge our present understanding of, and attitudes towards, childbirth and its psychological interpretation.

CONCLUSION

Pain is multidimensional and true understanding cannot be approached without considering its psychological facets alongside its physical manifestation. However the belief that pain has a psychological and emotional dimension is a relatively new idea, encapsulated by the theories of Melzack & Wall in 1965 which have barely been opposed by the medical fraternity and social scientists since.

The search for safe analgesia in labour has been a preoccupation of the medical profession, and has been encouraged by women's groups since the turn of the last century. The phenomenon of approaching labour pain as a positive and enlightening experience as opposed to a negatively viewed affliction has split the opinions of women, and the midwifery and medical professions, to the extent that in modern times the issues often become polarized and the needs of individual women no longer receive the focus that they deserve.

Studies of women's experience of their labours demonstrate that women generally do not focus on the issue of pain but tend to see it in the broader context of how supported they feel by their companions and attendants, how much choice they are given particularly in non-emergency situations and how in control they feel of unfolding events (including ability to cope without recourse to pharmacological analgesia, and access to pain-relieving drugs). Although some women report excruciating pain, the amount of pain generally bears little relationship to women's overall satisfaction with the labour and birth experience.

Major influences on the way women perceive labour pain are their cultural heritage, childbirth education (depending on its focus), the type of labour they

Useful resources

The best resource for midwives wishing to increase their knowledge about the psychology of pain in labour is to talk to women who have given birth.

have (particularly its length), the support they receive from attendants, the place of birth and the attitudes of attending health professionals.

ANNOTATED BIBLIOGRAPHY

Clement S (ed) 1998 Psychological perspectives on pregnancy and childbirth. Churchill Livingstone, Edinburgh

The authors of this book concentrate on particular aspects of the childbirth experience in depth rather than in breadth. Topics relevant to psychological issues include choice, control and decision making in labour, teenage motherhood and having a home birth. A problem-orientated approach is avoided (so there is no chapter on depression); rather the emphasis is on what can be done to prevent problems and promote health. Much of the emphasis of the chapters is on women's experiences and many of the authors are primary researchers.

Moore S 1997 Understanding pain and its relief in labour. Churchill Livingstone, London

The chapters in this book relevant to the psychology of pain in labour explore the psychosocial aspects of pain, a definition of pain and how it is measured, the cultural experience of pain and women's experiences of care by midwives. Themes which stand out include the need for culturally aware research and care from health professionals, the need for both women and health professionals to be aware of the complexity of pain sensation, labour environment and individual coping strategies, personality and pain perception and how care by midwives influences a woman's experience of labour.

Niven CA 1995 Psychological care for families. Butterworth Heinemann, Oxford

Kate Niven divides her book into sections; the second section covers birth and the issues addressed include stress and anxiety, pain, preparation, coping and social support. The author is a lecturer in psychology with a particular interest in childbirth and is an articulate assessor of research into the psychology of labour. Her conclusions are highly relevant to midwifery practice.

Raphael-Leff J 1991 Psychological processes of childbearing. Chapman and Hall, London.

Part five of Joan Raphael-Leff's discourse on psychological issues of childbearing deals with the preparation for and the experience of labour and birth. She expounds her theme of women being 'Facilitators' or 'Regulators'; Facilitators she defines as women who desire a natural birth in a private atmosphere and

Regulators as women who approach birth as a 'painful crisis which she intends to endure with minimal discomfort and maximum control' (p 241). The psychological effects of non-intervention and intervention on women during the birth process are examined.

Thomas P 1998 Every birth is different: women's experiences in their own words. Headline, London.

As the title suggests, women's accounts of their birth experience in their own words form the substance of this book. Inevitably emotional, psychological and cultural issues receive in-depth subjective analysis. The concepts of power, control and autonomy of both the women and the health professionals involved in their care receive attention, and the women describe vividly how different aspects of the birth environment affected their ability to deal with pain in both positive and negative ways.

REFERENCES

Bevis R 1984 Anaesthesia in midwifery. Baillière Tindall, London

Carter J, Duriez T 1986 With child: birth through the ages. Mainstream, Edinburgh

Chamberlain G, Wraight A, Crawley P 1997 Home births: the report of the 1994 confidential enquiry by the National Birthday Trust Fund. Parthenon Publishing Group, Carnforth, Lancs

Davies J, Hey E, Reid W et al 1996 Prospective regional study of planned home births. British Medical Journal 313: 1302–1306

Department of Health 1993 Report of the Expert Maternity Group. HMSO, London, p 8

Dick Read G 1943 Childbirth without fear. William Heinemann Medical, London pp 1, 9

Goldsmith J 1990 Childbirth wisdom. East West Health Books, Brookline, MA

Green JM, Coupland VA, Kitzinger JV 1998 Great expectations. Books for Midwives Press, Hale, Cheshire

Halldorsdottir S, Karlsdottir SI 1996 Journeying through labour and delivery: perceptions of women who have given birth. Midwifery 12: 48–61

Hillan EM 1992 Research and audit: women's views of caesarean section. In: Roberts H (ed) Women's health matters. Routledge, London, ch 9, pp 157–175

Hutton E 1994 What women want. British Journal of Midwifery 2: 608–611

Jowitt M 1993 Childbirth unmasked. Peter Wooller, Craven Arms, Shropshire

Kitzinger S 1997 Birth pain. MIDIRS Midwifery Digest 7: 331–333

Klaus MH, Kennell JH 1997 The doula: an essential ingredient of childbirth rediscovered. Acta Paediatrica 86: 1034–1036

McCourt C, Page L 1996 Report on the evaluation of one-to-one midwifery. Thames Valley University, London

Melzack R, Wall PD 1965 Pain mechanisms; a new theory. Science 150: 971–979

Melzack R, Wall P 1988 The challenge of pain. Penguin, London

Melzack R, Taenzer P, Feldman P, Kinch RA 1981 Labour is still painful after prepared childbirth training. Canadian Medical Association Journal 125: 357–363

Morrin NA 1997 Midwifery care in the first stage of labour. In: Sweet BR, Tiran D (eds) Mayes midwifery. Baillière Tindall, London, ch 29, pp 355–384

O'Driscoll K, Meagher D 1993 Active management of labour. Mosby, London

Office for National Statistics 1997 Birth statistics. Series FM1. HMSO, London

Ogden J 1996 Health psychology: a textbook. Open University Press, Milton Keynes

Rajan L 1993 Perceptions of pain and pain relief in labour: the gulf between experience and observation. Midwifery 9: 136–145

Ranta P, Jouppila P, Jouppila R 1996 The intensity of pain in grand multiparas. Acta Obstetrica et Gynecologica Scandinavica 75: 250–254

Rich A 1986 Of woman born. Virago, London

Rowley MJ, Hensley MJ, Brinsmead MW, Wlodarczyk JH 1995 Continuity of care by a midwife team versus routine care during pregnancy and birth: a randomised trial. Medical Journal of Australia 163: 289–293

Scopesi A, Zanobini M, Carossino P 1997 Childbirth in different cultures: psychophysical reactions of women delivering in US, German, French and Italian hospitals. Journal of Reproductive and Infant Psychology 15(1): 9–30

Simkin P 1995 Psychologic and other non-pharmacologic techniques. In: Bonica JJ, Mcdonald JS (eds) Principles and practices of obstetric analgesia and anesthesia. Williams and Wilkins, Baltimore, MD

Wetering M, Eskes TK 1988 Labour pain: a comparison of parturients in a Dutch and an American teaching hospital. Obstetrics and Gynaecology 71: 541–544

5

Sociocultural aspects of pain

Caroline Squire

KEY ISSUES

- ◆ Technology and childbirth
- ◆ Stereotyping
- ◆ Culture and pain

INTRODUCTION

Pain is a major feature of everyday life and is often related to injury and disease as a signal to indicate that something is wrong. Morris (1991) considers that pain is as elemental as fire or ice and that experience and construction of pain is decisively shaped or modified by individual human minds and by specific human cultures. He postulates that:

Medicine, in fact, because of its dominant position in our culture, tends automatically to suppress or to overpower all the other voices that offer us a different understanding of pain including voices of dissent within medicine (Morris 1991).

Helman (1990) makes the following propositions:

- ◆ Not all social or cultural groups may respond to pain in the same way.
- ◆ How people perceive and respond to pain, both in themselves and in others, can be largely influenced by their cultural background.
- ◆ How, and whether, people communicate their pain to health professionals and to others can also be influenced by social and cultural factors.

These propositions will be considered in this chapter in relation to the concept of pain. In doing so, the term 'culture' will be related to women and

61

our position in society as well as in a cross-cultural context. Biomedicine (western scientific medicine) will be considered as a sociocultural system in itself (Hahn & Kleinman 1983) and the experiences of women and their pain in childbirth will be situated and analysed within this framework. Finally, the concept of stereotyping will be discussed and how it impinges upon midwifery practice.

TECHNOLOGY AND CHILDBIRTH

Since publication of the Winterton Report (House of Commons 1992) and the 'Changing Childbirth' report (Department of Health 1993), great emphasis has been placed on the concept of woman-centred practice. However, the medicalization of birth and growth in science and technology has led towards fragmented practice, with births occurring in hospitals and an increase in interventions such as caesarean sections and instrumental deliveries and the use of the epidural for pain relief. Perceptions of pain experienced by women as well as perceptions of the efficacy of pain relief differ between women (Melzack 1984, Niven & Gijsbers 1984, Wraight 1993). Niven (1992) points out that studies of this kind have been carried out in hospital settings and it may be that labour pain is less intense when women give birth in familiar surroundings and are accompanied by staff with whom they have established a close relationship. With this in mind, it seems appropriate to explore theories concerning the effects of science and technology.

Oakley (1984) would argue that there are important parallels between medical and social ideologies of womanhood and that the theoretical foundations of patriarchy lie in the manipulation of woman's biology to constitute their inferiority. Hahn & Kleinman (1983) assert that biomedicine is a sociocultural system in itself because, as an artefact of human society, it sits within a cultural framework of values, premises and problematics, explicitly and implicitly taught by the communications of social interaction and then enacted in a social division of labour in institutional settings. With this in mind, it is not difficult to see how women's pain in childbirth has been captured and medicalized.

Renee Descartes was a seventeenth century philosopher and considered to be the source of the so-called Cartesian split between body and mind. This was an era of scientific discovery that produced the notion of a mechanistic universe which could be controlled by technology. This mind–body dualism has been deemed to have led to the metaphor of the body-as-machine (Helman 1990). Davis-Floyd (1987) has further argued that consideration of the body as a machine removed the body from the control of religion and placed it under the auspices of science. Men dominated the world of science as they do now and established the prototype of the machine as male, with the female viewed as a deviation from the norm, defective and unpredictable because it is influenced greatly by nature. As such, the female body needs protection from itself and manipulation when it goes wrong and Davis-Floyd (1987) would argue this to be the philosophical basis of modern obstetrics, the notion that culture (technology) controls nature. Furthermore, she suggests that many of the rituals of obstetrics also transmit some of society's most basic values to the woman giving birth. These include her powerlessness in the face of patriarchy, the need for medicine to control her body and her dependence on science and technology which, together, override and subsume individual beliefs and meanings.

Clearly this type of cultural message is much more likely to be transmitted in a hospital environment. As Kitzinger (1992) writes:

> *Whereas the traditional mode of childbirth places the women in the centre of the unfolding drama, modern childbirth involves advanced and sophisticated technology and cumbersome equipment, compared to which the labouring woman seems dwarfed and insignificant ... The ceremony of wiring up a woman in labour gives her the message that her body is not to be trusted and that it is in constant danger of malfunction.*

In a similar vein, the epidural, while providing effective anaesthesia for many women, also performs the function of immobilizing women in labour, necessitates an intravenous infusion and continuous electronic fetal heart rate monitoring. Apart from pain-relieving purposes, epidurals are strongly advised for such 'complications' as multiple and breech births. Here, the conceptualization of the passive, defective female requiring to be controlled is complete. Arney (1982) argues that pain relief is, in itself, a way of exerting control over women. With the arrival of the epidural, the groans and screams of women in the throes of labour are no longer so apparent. When they are, how many times have midwives heard comments from other midwives or obstetricians or anaesthetists such as: 'that women needs an epidural!' They do not know the woman and can have no appreciation of the dynamics taking place within the birthing room, yet they have made a judgement without knowledge or consultation with the woman concerned – she is marginal and needs controlling for her own good and that of her fetus.

Rajan's (1993) research concerning perceptions of pain and pain relief in labour reveals disparity between women and professionals. Non-pharmacological methods tended not to be included as pain-relieving techniques by the majority of obstetricians and anaesthetists, and members of each professional group tended to give primary consideration to those methods which fell within their own remit to administer. The implication was a view of the labouring woman limited by the boundaries of the individual's expertise or involvement and procluded any form of holistic practice.

The 'Changing Childbirth' report (Department of Health 1993) was underpinned by the concept of 'woman-centredness', where a woman is the focus of practice and her needs are paramount in decision making. However, institutions like the National Health Service are hierarchical and made up of tiers of professions each with their own codes of practice and agendas. It is easy to see how a woman can be marginalized when she becomes the centre of competing ideologies and professional practices. In a study by Green (1993) expectations and actual experiences of pain were considered in a prospective study of 825 responses to postal questionnaires and it was worrying that 10% of the respondents felt pressure from staff not to use drugs and a further 7% felt pressure to use drugs. What agendas were at play here? Were the results due to poor communication and not listening to women, were they due to professional expertise or were staff using their own frameworks to pass judgements? The reasons are unknown but it is important for midwives to be aware of these dynamics to prevent marginalization and objectification of women. Women seem to want, among others, control of self and circumstances (Department of Health 1993; Halldorsdottir & Karlsdottir 1996) and it is crucial that midwives, acting as skilled companions, fulfil these needs.

Doctors, and to some extent midwives, are educated using a biomedical framework. Here, theories of pain 'concentrate upon its neurophysiological aspects, both in diagnosis and treatment ... rather than seeing it as moulded and shaped both by the individual and their particular socio-cultural context' (Bendelow & Williams 1995). Thus, the obvious answer to pain is to cure it. This sits firmly within the dominant scientific paradigm and explains remarks like 'if you have a toothache, you need pain relief – like childbirth, it is painful, so have an epidural or book your caesarean birth'. In our technological age, many women are booking caesarean sections or wanting planned epidurals. Anthropologists would want to consider why this has happened and might suggest that women have lost confidence in their ability to give birth unaided (Symonds & Hunt 1996) due to the power of the professionals who have conceptualized birth as pathology where medical intervention is necessary to ensure a safe outcome.

A Cartesian mind–body dualism can be perceived through women's experiences of pain and would be closely related to control of self and circumstances. Women may report being overpowered with each contraction, going mad, losing control and feeling helpless (Halldorsdottir & Karlsdottir 1996). Martin's (1989) study revealed the same with women reporting that their subjective feelings were marginalized in favour of their objective scientifically measured bodily responses. Rajan (1993) also reported that there were a significant number of instances in her study in which perceptions of the effectiveness of analgesia differed widely between the women and the professionals who attended them, particularly where the woman felt her pain was not helped by the method, although the professional believed it was. Rajan cites pethidine in particular where there were frequent instances of women complaining that not only was the drug not helpful during labour as it took away their sense of control, but also one of the side-effects where it was administered too late in the first stage of labour often disadvantaged the establishment of breastfeeding.

Midwives need to consider a woman in an holistic sense in order to recognize her individual experience. Rajan (1993) continues by suggesting that discrepancies between women's and midwives' perceptions of the efficacy of pain relief is that midwives are comparing each woman's labour with others they have attended. Therefore frames of reference will be different, which may result in stereotypical practice and impoverishment of the individual woman's birth experience.

STEREOTYPING

Stereotyping is the use of internal models and sets of assumptions to think about and interact with other people (Green et al 1990). Midwives and other professionals will use them to make generalizations about groups of women based on literature, the media and, sometimes, peer pressure. Such stereotyping may promote crude, ineffective practice as well as, at a macrolevel, inappropriate social policy or provision of maternity services.

Green et al (1990) have published a research paper concerning stereotypes of childbearing women from a larger study of expectations and experiences of pain in labour. How many times have midwives heard colleagues discussing 'the NCT type' or the fact that uneducated, working-class women expect to suffer in childbirth and do not need information? The 'NCT type' would typically be described as well educated and middle class, has read all the books and is prone to postnatal depression when her overly high expectations are not met. Green and her colleagues found that these stereotypes were not supported in several respects. First, women of different education levels were equally likely to subscribe to the ideal of avoiding drugs in labour. Second, the NCT type wanted to be and was relatively well informed about labour and birth and wanted control of decision making. Related to the larger study (Green 1993), high expectations were not exclusive to better educated women, nor were such expectations found to be disadvantageous. Indeed, they were found to be instrumental in achieving positive outcomes. Clearly, midwives can feel confident in promoting such expectations.

With respect to the stereotype of the less-educated woman, Green et al (1990) found that she was just as interested as her better educated counterpart with the concept of birth as fulfilling. Furthermore, although she had lower expectations of being in control of her environment and decision making, nevertheless she still wanted to be involved. Midwives need to view women as individuals rather than use stereotypes. Women, overwhelmingly, need to be central to the decision-making process.

Negative stereotypes were found in Bowler's (1993) small-scale ethnographic research concerning women of Asian descent which were worrying because they were unkind and seemed to reveal individual and institutional racism. For example, in terms of communication, some midwives assumed that none of the Asian women spoke or understood English, whereas the researchers found that many spoke a little but were shy and understood broadly what was said to them. As a consequence of communication problems, women were often perceived as rather stupid and some midwives felt unrewarded because they felt unable to develop a trusting relationship with them. Bowes & Domokos (1996) in their research concerning muted voices of Pakistani women and maternity care, quote one of their informants, an articulate woman who usually wore western clothes but wore Punjabi dress when attending the antenatal clinic:

> *I will wear these clothes, and open my mouth later on to shock people –*
> *you know, shock white people, because they think this is an idiot sitting*
> *there wearing these clothes.*

With regard to pain, 'making a fuss about nothing' was a recurring expression quoted from some midwives in Bowler's paper. Others included attention-seeking, making too much noise, unnecessary fuss because of low pain thresholds.

Bowes & Domokos (1996) also found that many of their informants had not attended parent education sessions because, like many women, of difficulties in using public transport and long waiting times in the clinic, especially when they had small children with them. One of the informants said that the midwife during her labour was very punitive towards her because she had not attended parent education classes and refused to give her pain relief because she had not been taught how to breathe or use the gas. Windsor-Richards & Gillies (1988), in a study comparing racial grouping and women's experiences of giving birth in hospital, found that Asian women were more likely to have pain relief administered to them without discussion or explanation, which is abusive.

It seems clear that there are serious problems of communication here, a theme that has recurred throughout the literature (Bharj 1995, Health Education Authority 1995, Schott & Henley 1996). Furthermore, Bowler (1993) attended the births of six Asian and four white women and did not find that the Asian women made a greater deal of noise. It is a key theme of this chapter that midwives need to avoid negative stereotyping and assess women of whatever background as individuals with personal needs and wishes.

Using negative stereotypes of minority women of colour is racist, although as Williams' (Bradby 1995) study of the history of the Irish in Britain shows, discrimination is not dependent on colour. However, colour has been said to be the greatest single factor that governs society's attitude (Rack 1991). Racism has been defined as 'prejudice combined with power' (Neile 1997) and implies a belief in the superiority of a race which leads to unfair discriminatory acts. These discriminatory acts may be at a national policy level, an institutional level or on a personal basis.

In the UK, the Race Relations Act of 1976 forbids discrimination against a person on grounds of race which includes colour, race, nationality, ethnic or national origins (Schott & Henley 1996). It is outside the remit here to consider racism fully. Suffice to say, it behoves all midwives to be self aware to ensure we do not practise in a discriminatory way.

CULTURE AND PAIN

Labour is very painful for most women. There are only a very few women who experience a natural painless birth. However, how each woman is able to cope with it depends on factors which might include cultural attitude towards the normalcy and conduct of birth, expectations of how a woman should act in labour and the degree and quality of social support (Lauderdale & Greener 1995). Physiological factors are important too, and would include the quality and frequency of contractions, the size and position of the fetus, and the use of painful obstetric interventions (Bonica 1995).

Cultural attitudes towards the normalcy and conduct of birth clearly differ. As Jordan (1993) explains:

> *What is of interest is not whether women do or do not experience pain, but rather what sort of an 'object' pain becomes in different systems: is it highlighted or discounted?*

Jordan has written a sensitive and insightful account of childbirth in Yucatan, Holland, Sweden and the USA. In her fieldwork, she concludes that the experience of pain is more visible in delivery suites in the USA than it is in Holland, Sweden or Yucatan and that the expectations engendered by the local conception of birth influence the level of pain display and experience. Sweden and Holland, of course, are developed countries but Jordan would argue that conceptions of birth are different. In the USA analgesia is available but the woman must convince her nurse that she needs it by an appropriate display of pain experience.

Similar findings were found in Rajan's (1993) study, which revealed that some women found their experiences of pain were not recognized by professionals. This was perhaps because different frameworks were used which meant that midwives and doctors were not focusing on an individual's subjective experience and, thereby, objectifying her, or because pain relief was not judged to be in the woman's or the baby's best interest.

In Sweden, pharmacological pain relief is also available but Jordan (1993) found that women do not have to convince their midwives that they need it because that decision is considered to belong to the woman and not the midwife. In Holland, Jordan contends that Dutch women and midwives view birth as a natural process and interference, which would include pharmacological pain relief, would be considered inappropriate if possible. Van Hollen (1994), however, critiques Jordan's work by stating that it reveals little variation in beliefs and practices associated with birth within a given culture. Thus, little attention has been paid to unequal social divisions based on, for example, class and gender, which may impinge upon local conceptions of birth and, therefore, on the experience of pain.

In a study of women and childbearing in a village in Uttar Pradesh, India, Jeffrey et al (1989) consider childbearing within the context of family relationships, household economy and stratification of society. In a patriarchal, agrarian society, where a woman is expected to belong to her husband's family, childbirth is considered a polluting condition which takes place in her husband's social setting. In this study, there were no remedies for reducing the pain but plenty to stimulate pain because it was thought that intense pain is necessary to ensure a speedy delivery. Expression of pain was thought shameful here; pain should be accepted as part of the birth process. This did not mean that women did not have painful births though and quotations from the women testified to this.

Of course, assessment of pain through self reporting is fraught with problems. 'Pain is what the subject says hurts' may at first seem logical, but clearly denies possible traits of stoicism, exaggeration and other cultural variables and sits firmly within a reductionist scientific discourse.

Language is used to communicate to another whether one is experiencing pain and is part of the cultural expression of individuals. Culture may be transmitted through language verbally or in the written form. If a culture tends to prohibit pain expression, then expression may not occur in the form of language. Waddie (1996) poses the possibility that if clinicians depend solely on language to establish or confirm the existence of pain, then it is possible that the aim is not to relieve the pain but to silence the client. This may sound contentious, but consider the midwife in Bowes & Domokos' (1996) research who did not administer pain relief to the Asian woman who had not attended parent education sessions. Clearly, non-verbal communication and meanings of pain must be considered in assessment.

Harrison et al (1996) wonders whether sharing a mother-tongue affects how closely patients and nurses agree when rating the patient's pain, worry and knowledge. In this small-scale study, it was found that only nurses sharing a mother-tongue with the patient provided pain ratings which correlated significantly with those of their patients. Again, this has implications for interpretation and communication.

Cultural and educational influences on the pain of childbirth were considered by Weisenberg & Caspi (1989). Their study examined the reactions to the pain of childbirth among women from a middle eastern as opposed to a western family of origin in terms of the influences of culture, education and family of origin on the verbal ratings of pain and pain behaviour during childbirth. It was found, as expected, that all women rated the pain as high but middle eastern women gave higher ratings of pain and demonstrated more pain behaviour, particularly those with less education. The authors conclude:

It is likely that educational influences can change the original contribution of family of origin on the reaction to pain.

Furthermore, Weissenberg & Caspi (1989) considered that participation in parent education sessions led to a significant reduction in pain behaviour although pain ratings remained unchanged. While one would welcome the apparent endorsement that parent education might be useful in reducing anxiety and fear in labour, midwives need to be careful to remember that cultural groups are not homogeneous and nor are women. Therefore, the value of comparing cultural groups would need to be questioned and women considered in terms of being individuals in order to avoid the dangers of stereotyping.

'Poststructuralism' is a theory of the relationship between language, subjectivity, social organizations and power (Weedon 1987, Price & Cheek 1996) and is a useful perspective when considering the reporting of pain. How a patient is asked to self report pain, to give meaning to pain, is dependent on how pain is constructed by individuals, including health professionals (Price & Cheek 1996). It may be that, as mentioned in Rajan's paper (1993), midwives and doctors focus on a woman's pain in relation to their experience of other women's pain and fail to focus on first, the woman herself rather than the pain, and second, the woman as an individual and, therefore what she brings to their interactions. Such dynamics, of course, require the professionals to be aware not only of themselves but also of their own professional culture and education which may influence their thinking and interpretations. Poststructuralist theorists do not discount the biomedical paradigm; they seek recognition of other discourses because they advocate plurality of meaning and possibilities. Poststructuralism, then, seems a useful framework to help those midwives who are seeking more woman-centred approaches to the conceptualization of women and their pain in childbirth.

Box 5.1 gives suggestions for midwifery practice.

CONCLUSION

The chapter has attempted to consider that as midwives we are a heterogeneous group, as are women and their families. In order to practise sensitively and insightfully, we need to have a deep understanding of women in society and the culture of medicine, in particular obstetrics, and also the

---

Box 5.1 Suggestions for midwifery practice

◆ It is important not to view groups of women as a uniform, homogeneous group. This will lead to the use of negative stereotypes

◆ Women need to be at the centre of the decision-making process

◆ Women are different. Therefore, midwives need to educate themselves in the sociocultural context of women and childbirth

◆ Midwives need to be self aware of ourselves as, largely, women and as midwives. Only when we understand our own frameworks can we begin to understand other women so that they can truly be the subject of practice

◆ Senior midwives who are involved in policy making must ensure they recognize that women are the only people who can identify their own personal needs

◆ Senior midwives and administrators must be aware of institutionalized assumptions and discriminatory practices which are racist and eliminate them

◆ Senior midwives and administrators need to ensure the following are provided:

  — linkworkers as promoted in the Asian Mother and Baby Campaign in the 1980s

  — language-specific leaflets and information

  — parent education specific to client group needs

  — inservice education or funding for study day/courses to promote an understanding of the differences of client groups and their needs

  — a copy of The Commission for Racial Equality's Code of Practice 1994 for every midwife (CRE 1994)

relationship between women and technological and scientific discourses. It may be said that women from different cultural backgrounds are doubly disadvantaged and it is, therefore, vital that midwives do not practise in an ethnocentric manner and make every effort to become culturally aware. Pain and its meanings are important concepts to have an understanding of and will go part of the way towards helping different women achieve what they want when they give birth to their children.

ANNOTATED BIBLIOGRAPHY

Cheung NF 1994 Pain in normal labour. A comparison of experiences in southern China and Scotland. Midwives Chronicle June: 212–216

This is an interesting article in which a midwife makes a comparison of women's experiences of birth in southern China and Scotland. She argues that cultural background has a key role in the perception of pain and pain tolerance and this can be altered by rationalization.

Fordham M, Dunn V 1994 Alongside the person in pain. Baillière Tindall, London, especially ch 3

Chapter 3, 'The nature and meaning of pain', is taken from an excellent book, which, although it does not focus on childbirth, nonetheless would constitute useful background reading in order to understand more fully the concept of pain. The aspects considered here include the neurophysiology of pain, the experience and expression of pain, the meaning of pain and self knowledge.

Moore S (ed) 1997 Understanding pain and its relief in labour. Churchill Livingstone, London, especially chs 2, 4, 6

Chapter 2, 'Defining pain', is written by the editor who is a midwife. The specific aspects of this chapter which are particularly interesting include perception of pain, purpose of pain, phenomena of labour, explaining pain and types of pain. 'Psychology of pain' (Chapter 4) is also written by the editor. The specific aspects of this chapter which are particularly useful to the reader include pain behaviour, labour environment, psychology, pregnancy, childbirth and midwifery care, pain perception, coping strategies and the effect of carers and psychoanalysis and childbirth. Chapter 6, 'A cultural experience of pain', considers an introduction to the cultural influences on the concept of pain. As such, the key aspects looked at include effective communication, provision of maternity care, stereotypes, a culture of pain, culture and labour and cultural considerations for midwifery practice. Issues surrounding experiences of women from a particular ethnic group are identified, as well as key aspects for midwifery practice.

Wagner M 1997 Pursuing the birth machine. Ace Graphics, Camperdown, Australia, especially ch 6

This chapter, 'Technology for birth: a consensus meeting in Fortaleza, Brazil', considers aspects of birth which have been taken over by science and technology. Pages 153–158, in particular, consider the use of pain relief in technological births.

REFERENCES

Arney WR 1982 Power and the profession of obstetrics. Sociology of Health and Illness 4(1)

Bendelow GA, Williams SJ 1995 Transcending the dualisms: towards a sociology of pain. Sociology of Health and Illness 17(12): 139–165

Bharj K 1995 Providing midwifery care in a multi-cultural society. British Journal of Midwifery 3: 271–276

Bonica J 1995 The nature of the pain in parturition. In: Bonica J, Macdonald JS (eds) Principles of obstetric analgesia and anaesthesia, 2nd edn. Williams and Wilkins, Baltimore, pp 243–273

Bowes AM, Domokos TM 1996 Pakistani women and maternity care: raising muted voices. Sociology of Health and Illness 18(1): 45–65

Bowler I 1993 Stereotypes of women of Asian descent in midwifery: some evidence. Midwifery 9: 7–16

Bradby H 1995 Ethnicity: not a black and white issue. A research note. Sociology of Health and Illness 17(3): 405–417

Commission for Racial Equality 1994 Race relations code of practice. Maternity services. CRE, London

Davis-Floyd R 1987 The technological model of birth. Journal of American Folklore 100: 479–495

Department of Health 1993 Report of the Expert Advisory Committee. Chair Baroness Cumberledge. HMSO, London

Green JM 1993 Expectations and experiences of pain in labour. Birth 20(2): 65–72

Green JM, Kitzinger JV, Coupland VA 1990 Stereotypes of childbearing women: a look at some evidence. Midwifery 6: 125–132

Hahn RA, Kleinman A 1983 Biomedical practice and anthropological theory: frameworks and directions. Annual Review of Anthropology 12: 305–333

Halldorsdottir S, Karlsdottir S 1996 Journeying through labour and delivery: perceptions of women who have given birth. Midwifery 12(2): 48–61

Harrison A, Busabir AA, Obeid Al-Kaabi A, Khalid Al-Awadi H 1996 Does sharing a mother-tongue affect how closely patients and nurses agree when rating the patients' pain, worry and knowledge? Journal of Advanced Nursing 24: 229–235

Health Education Authority 1995 Black and minority ethnic groups in England. Health and lifestyles. HEA Publishing, London

Helman C 1990 Culture, health and illness, 2nd edn. Wright, London, pp 147, 159

House of Commons 1992 Second Report of the Social Select Committee. Chair Sir N Winterton. HMSO, London

Jeffery P, Jeffery R, Lyons A 1989 Labour pains and labour power. Zed Press, London, p 105

Jordan B 1993 Birth in four cultures. Waveland, Prospect Heights, Illinois, p 52

Kitzinger S 1992 Ourselves as mothers. Doubleday, London, pp 142–143

Lauderdale J, Greener DL 1995 Transcultural nursing care of the child-bearing family. In: Andrews M, Boyle J (eds) Transcultural concepts in nursing care, 2nd edn. JB Lippincott, Philadelphia, ch 3, p 110

Martin E 1989 The woman in the body. Open University Press, Milton Keynes

Melzack R 1984 The myth of painless childbirth. Pain 19: 321–337

Morris D 1991 The culture of pain. University of California Press, London, pp 1, 2

Neile E 1997 Control for Black and Ethnic minority women: a meaningless pursuit. In: Kirkham M, Perkins E (eds) Reflections on midwifery. Baillière Tindall, London, p 115

Niven CA 1992 Psychological care for families: before, during and after birth. Butterworth-Heinemann, Oxford, p 46

Niven C, Gijsbers K 1984 Obstetric and non-obstetric factors related to labour pain. Journal of Reproductive and Infant Psychology 2: 61–78

Oakley A 1984 Doctor knows best. 3.9 Health and disease. A reader. Open University Press, Miltan Keynes, p 171

Price K, Cheek J 1996 Exploring the nursing role in pain management from a post-structuralist perspective. Journal of Advanced Nursing 24: 899–904

Rack P 1991 Race, culture and mental disorders. Routledge, London

Rajan L 1993 Perceptions of pain and pain relief in labour: the gulf between experience and observation. Midwifery 9: 136–145

Schott J, Henley A 1996 Culture, religion and childbearing in a multi-racial society. Butterworth-Heinemann, Oxford

Symonds A, Hunt SC 1996 The midwife and society. Macmillan, Basingstoke, p 94

Van Hollen C 1994 Review article. Perspectives on the anthropology of birth. Culture, Medicine and Psychiatry 18: 501–512

Waddie N 1996 Language and pain expression. Journal of Advanced Nursing 23: 868–872

Weedon C 1987 Feminist practices and post-structuralist theory. Basil Blackwell, New York

Weisenberg M, Caspi Z 1989 Cultural and educational influences on pain of childbirth. Journal of Pain and Symptom Management 4(1): 13–19

Windsor-Richards K, Gillies PA 1988 Racial groupings and women's experience of giving birth in hospital. Midwifery 4: 171–176

Wraight A 1993 Coping with pain. In: Chamberlain G, Wraight A, Steer P (eds) Pain and its relief in childbirth. Churchill Livingstone, London, ch 8

6

Relief of pain and discomfort in labour: a moral and legal perspective

Carmel Bagness

KEY ISSUES

- ◆ Autonomy and control
- ◆ Informed choice and consent
- ◆ Effective decision making
  A voluntary decision
  What is competence?
  How much information is appropriate?
- ◆ Accountability for practice
  Record keeping
  Accountability
  New therapies and strategies for relief of pain
- ◆ Administration of medication

INTRODUCTION

One of the main issues concerning many pregnant women on the challenge of labour is the management of anticipated pain and discomfort. The variety of choices for relief are increasing constantly, making it necessary for women to make decisions about their preferences. The challenge for midwives is to provide optimum care which will enable women to feel satisfied with the experience. One of the problems with measuring satisfaction is that, just as each woman is an individual, so will her experience be unique and her measurement of a satisfactory labour may be very different to that of the midwife's perception of the success of the event. Even when the outcome may not have been happy, or as expected, the woman should still be able to feel satisfied that her needs for pain relief were met.

The focus of this chapter will be on the ethical and legal concepts which should enable the midwife to facilitate the woman's positive experience with the use of pain relief during labour. Details of the various methods and strategies available have been discussed elsewhere and will be referred to collectively here.

Individual moral codes are established by past events, life experiences, thoughts and actions and should not be underestimated when considering influences on decision making. They have been formed through a lifetime of individual and diverse experiences. Consequently different midwives and different mothers (and their partners) may have similar or different values and beliefs about aspects of life, and as such all practices should reflect a respect for such differences.

The now well-quoted 'Changing Childbirth Report' (Department of Health 1993) was clear in its expectations of the midwifery profession and reflected the need to concentrate more attention on individual needs. It also went further than previous reports by asserting women's right to be in control of their pregnancy and childbirth, advocating that the midwife and woman work in partnership to achieve decided outcomes. The importance of this particular concept of partnership is that it advocates the provision of services that offer the mother choice, control and continuity for childbirth (Department of Health 1993) and should provide the midwife with the satisfaction of being 'with women' and facilitating a positive experience wherever possible. As will be seen, this is vital if ethical principles of autonomy and respect for that autonomy, as well as informed consent and choice, are to be upheld to the woman's satisfaction.

Distinction is not made in the text between primigravid and multigravid women; suffice to say that all women should be supported according to their individual needs. The focus of current discussion is very much on the mother and midwife, however acknowledgement should also be made regularly to the woman's partner who may play a significant role in any decisions taken, choices made and the assertion of her needs and expectations, particularly when she is in labour.

The midwife, as well as having moral duties, also has to function effectively within the legal framework of practice. The main considerations here are with accountability and scope of practice, balancing the needs and expectations of women, with the midwife's own needs for autonomous, safe practice – to maintain a healthy partnership.

It must also be remembered that midwives are not only responsible for the mother but they have a duty to consider the well being of the fetus and baby when decisions are taken and acted on. This is particularly pertinent when contemplating the administration of medication during labour.

AUTONOMY AND CONTROL

In 1993 the International Confederation of Midwives (ICM) developed an International Code of Ethics for Midwives, and the first principle they proposed was that 'midwives respect a woman's informed right of choice and promote the woman's acceptance of responsibility for the outcomes of her choices' (International Confederation of Midwives 1994). The code was based on the ideology of mutual trust, respect and good relationships, and it reflected the expectations of 'Changing Childbirth' (Department of Health 1993) in focusing on the concept of women and midwives working together. In theory, few would disagree with this, however in practice it can be more difficult to achieve because of the diversity of mothers, midwives and the choices now available. Accordingly, it could be argued that both mothers and midwives have a responsibility to be fully aware of the options, choices and possible conflicts that may impinge on decision making and any subsequent practices.

In order for midwives to facilitate women's autonomous decisions about their labour, it is necessary that they should explore and understand the concept. This will inevitably involve the midwife having a sense of her own professional autonomy and personal assertiveness, as well as believing in the woman's. It includes an increased understanding of the woman's right to assert her needs and expectations and have them responded to in a responsible and dignified way that demonstrates her place in the midwife–mother partnership.

Beauchamp & Childress (1994) define autonomy as an ability to make informed decisions about one's life and take responsibility for those decisions, understanding the consequences and without (coercive or obstructive) controlling influences. For midwives, this involves being fully aware of their scope of practice and accountability for that practice, which includes understanding of the consequences of any action taken. It also encompasses the need for midwives to be able to professionally assert any concerns or needs they may have.

Controlling influences on practice are often related to individual perceptions, however these should be regarded as empowering, rather than coercive or obstructive. For example, one of the key factors for current practice is the need to maintain and develop acceptable strategies for continuity of care. Some midwives feel that the expectations for providing continuity in some schemes involves extensive commitment from them. This may be beyond previous expectations, leading to feelings of not being in control of practice which may significantly impinge on their own lives. A recent report by Sandell (1997) demonstrated that some of these fears were well founded and that such projects should be well supported and consider the needs of all those involved, facilitating a respect for the midwife's autonomy as well as the woman's. As a result of adequate consultation, they could then be viewed more positively in retaining and developing midwives' professional autonomy, otherwise they may have adverse effects on midwives' practice and well being, sometimes leading to burn-out and midwives leaving the profession (Sandell 1997).

With regard to women's autonomy, Schott (1994) suggests that one of the key factors in successful parenting is the need for women to have confidence in their abilities and decision-making skills. Consequently 'the way parents are cared for during pregnancy and childbirth is crucial in laying foundations of confidence and self-esteem' (Schott 1994).

The key issue for the midwife and mother has to be extensive open discussions, which consider flexible options regarding choices for pain relief. This has to begin during antenatal care, and forms a significant part of the necessity of building effective and positive relationships between women and midwives – effective communication, providing accurate and honest information, with appropriate listening to each other. This also implies the need to encourage women to be assertive in vocalizing their needs, with the midwife acting as advocate when necessary. The significance of mutual understanding and trust underpins the whole concept of individualized care and will lead to a stronger partnership, which should support safe autonomous practice for the woman and the midwife during pregnancy, childbirth and the postnatal period.

For some women, pregnancy and labour may be the first occasion when they have been faced with such decision making, consequently the experience may be frightening, challenging or daunting. Some may not feel or recognize a need to develop the necessary skills and may wish to transfer the responsibility to another, i.e. the midwife. In this situation midwives have two choices.

The midwife may choose to take a paternalistic view and 'help' the woman make her decisions. The consequences of this may be a lack of understanding from the midwife of the woman's real needs, because assumptions may be made in the process of this helping strategy. The outcome may be positive; however it may result in a negative experience, with the woman blaming the midwife – after all the midwife made the decision for her. This response can have far-reaching consequences, not just for the woman, who will eventually have to develop her decision-making skills, and may have to face that challenge with a new baby to care for as well. Such action by the midwife may do little for the profession, as the blame laid at the midwife may travel with the woman's story of her birth.

The alternative would be to recognize the need to develop the woman's understanding of her need to make decisions, *and take responsibility for them,* by enabling her to acquire the necessary skills, during her pregnancy. This can be achieved by encouraging the woman to question the choices available and check understanding, without being patronized. It also involves providing appropriate support so that she believes in her decisions, asserts her needs and has them listened to and respected. Producing accurate, understandable information and encouraging her to think about the options in a rational and reflective manner *before* labour is imminent are essential factors in increasing her autonomy and assertiveness. Further guidance is provided for midwives in the 'Guidelines for Professional Practice' (UKCC (United Kingdom Central Council for Nurses, Midwives and Health Visitors) 1996) publication.

Midwives are as concerned today as ever about being 'with woman' and the numerous recent developments in practice demonstrate an understanding of the importance of the woman feeling that she is in control of her birthing experience. In order to achieve this the woman has to be in a position to know the options available to her, give informed consent and believe that her autonomy is being respected. From personal experience the author has found that some midwives feel that in facilitating this they may lose some of their autonomy and control. Consequently it is necessary to maintain a balance so that both mothers and midwives feel that they can act autonomously and both have a sense of achievement and success. This should not be at the expense of either and it involves consideration of the concept of control and what that means.

For midwives, it may be an understanding that they retain control over their practice (e.g. by being involved in planning strategies), while adjusting former ideas about who should make individual decisions about a particular woman's needs. Having said that, some women may need encouragement to develop the skills necessary to appreciate their right to take control, make decisions and assume responsibility for those decisions.

Midwives are always accountable for their practice and occasionally this may conflict with the mother's wishes. The examples often quoted suggest situations where expectations may conflict with possible fetal well being. For example, the woman who is adamant in using the birthing pool when it is contraindicated. The midwife is responsible for the safety and well being of both mother and fetus (Jones 1994), and may feel unable to comply with her wishes. In practice, there are very few women who will put their fetus/baby at risk and often such conflicts arise because of inadequate communication causing misunderstandings, where the woman may have unrealistic expectations based on unsound information which should have been discussed antenatally. Consequently, the importance of effective communication cannot be emphasized enough in supporting autonomy for women and their midwives.

INFORMED CHOICE AND CONSENT

Informed choice and consent are key factors in practice and are a necessary part of the process of the partnership between women and midwives. Even though they should go hand in hand in practice, there is a significant difference which needs acknowledgement – choice is a moral expectation and right, whereas consent has a legal element and may be viewed differently, especially if problems arise.

It may be argued that in order to give informed consent to accepting proposed analgesia or any other treatment, the woman needs to know intimately the choices that are available to her. It is also worth noting that a significant majority of women are far more inquisitive antenatally and will make every attempt to investigate the choices and discuss them with their midwife/midwives. As with many issues, problems only arise when this process has not taken place, often because of incomplete understanding by the women and by midwives.

This may be related to women's perception of just how much control they may really have and how such perceptions are based on past experiences or hearsay. Consequently, the midwife should be aware of such influences and the need to persist in supporting the woman to become more autonomous. Women who have not had the opportunity to be autonomous and assertive may find it uncomfortable and unsettling initially; however with increased confidence and genuine support from midwives, they will realize the enhancement to their lives being in control can bring (Dickson 1992). The support provided by midwives should also facilitate the woman's right to reject certain or all methods offered and explore alternative strategies for achieving her needs in labour.

The essence of informed consent and choice for pain relief in labour involves open dialogue between midwife and mother, the partnership should begin early in the antenatal period, and even if the same midwife is not caring for the woman during labour she should feel adequately prepared and able to assert her needs to anyone. Gillon (1985) defines consent as a voluntary decision, made by a sufficiently competent and autonomous person on the basis of information, to accept a proposed course of action.

There are several elements of this concept to be considered in relation to pain relief in labour:

◆ a voluntary decision
◆ competence and accepting responsibility for the decision
◆ information giving.

A voluntary decision

A voluntary decision is one made where the person is not under the control of influences which may be viewed as coercive, persuasive or manipulative (Beauchamp & Childress 1994). Accordingly, midwives need to be aware of the circumstances and environment in which information is given to the women. Mander (1996) provides an interesting discussion regarding subtle coercion in the recommendations for the use of epidural analgesia for pain relief. She suggests that midwives and other health professionals are inevitably influenced by their own personal experience and may use that (often unintentionally) to place a certain emphasis on the advantages and/or disadvantages of procedures, regardless of other available evidence. Women will be influenced by a variety of factors, which is one reason why they need time antenatally to reflect on these options rather than attempting to assimilate all the information when in labour.

What is competence?

The majority of women are considered competent, however defining exactly what that means may be difficult. Beauchamp & Childress (1994) suggest a basic definition of an 'ability to perform a skill', but more specifically the criteria for that skill may vary enormously depending on the task in hand. Accordingly 'the competence to decide … is relative to the particular decision to be made' (Beauchamp & Childress 1994: p 134). It could be reasonably argued that women's competence to make decisions will be influenced by both internal and external forces. For women in labour, the pain and discomfort felt may significantly alter perceptions of needs. In practice this is seen with women who are determined antenatally that they would not have an epidural, but in labour change their minds. Ideally such decisions should be discussed in detail beforehand, offering time to reflect and support the idea of keeping options open. This gives women control over decisions, by allowing them to keep to original plans or change their minds. Experience suggests that some women who have adamant wishes antenatally may make these based on some rather than all the available information. Sometimes such a decision can be overlooked and may then lead to conflict when the woman is in labour, leaving the midwife unsure of how to proceed for fear of recriminations afterwards. Ethically, women should feel fully supported and in sufficient control to change their minds and accept the consequences of that decision at all times. The message here, as always, is about effective communication antenatally and in early labour.

How much information is appropriate?

As with all aspects of practice, the midwife needs to understand each woman, avoiding stereotyping assumptions and providing good information accordingly. Mander (1993) suggests that choices are only as good as the information provided, consequently if the midwife is concerned with good practice then only the best possible information or access to information for women is made available. This also involves being acutely aware of prejudices and conjectures that may have developed with practice about certain women's needs and expectations. All explanations should be in a manner that is intelligible to that woman, avoiding jargon and assessing understanding. All known benefits and risks should be clarified and possible alternatives suggested.

The timing of giving information regarding pain relief can be difficult. Many women will have been concerned about this throughout their pregnancy and will have investigated the alternatives for themselves. However some leave concerns about labour until nearer the estimated date of delivery. Some women may go into premature labour, others may not wish to discuss the matter, using statements like 'I'll wait and see'. Women who may be reluctant should be encouraged to discuss the reasons for their reluctance and the midwife may find that fear or unrealistic expectations may be the cause of their denial of future events. The midwife has the responsibility of striking a balance and should introduce the issue early, providing details of the alternatives. Managing pain can be a very sensitive issue and women need to explore all the issues with their birth partner and the midwife, before they can make informed decisions, and before they expect to be in labour (Reflective scenario 6.1).

Midwives should also take into consideration the multifactorial influences on decision making, such as culture, religious convictions, education, peer pressure, previous experience, etc. If midwives are to encourage autonomy in the women they meet, they should always encourage open discussion and flexible decision making – it should always be stressed that women may not know how they may react, even if they have had previous labours, as they are often different. If women believe that they are in control and have

---

Reflective scenario 6.1

Penny is a 17-year-old unsupported primigravida, who has had limited antenatal care and did not attend parent education classes – she 'reckoned they were boring'. She is in early labour, but refuses to discuss her options for pain relief and is adamant that she will manage with nothing. Her baby is lying in an occipitoposterior position and she has back-ache. Experience suggests that she may need some effective pain relief later and it may be a long labour.

What can the midwife do to support her and enable her to make some informed decisions about her impending labour?

options, they will feel better prepared and able to assert their needs and wishes with the midwife and others.

The factors involved in effective decision making and informed choice and consent throughout pregnancy, labour and the postnatal period are shown in Box 6.1.

ACCOUNTABILITY FOR PRACTICE

Midwives have a duty to practice within the legal frameworks which support registration with the UKCC and as such any practice involving relief of pain may be influenced by the power of that framework. The legal aspects considered here focus on the midwife's practice, in particular, record keeping, accountability and involvement in new therapies. The midwife should also be mindful of the role of the supervisor of midwives in providing support and advice for situations that may be potentially problematic, especially in anticipation of conflict. The administration of medication will be covered in the next section.

Record keeping

The competent practice of midwives involves the necessity to keep as contemporaneously as is reasonable detailed accurate and legible 'records of all observations, care given and medicine or other forms of pain relief' administered during practice (Rule 42: 18: UKCC 1998). The importance of

---

Box 6.1 Factors involved in effective decision making, informed choice and consent throughout pregnancy, labour and the postnatal period

◆ The midwife providing critically analysed, evidence based, up-to-date information which is easily understood by the mother

◆ The woman being enabled to understand, reflect on and absorb all the elements of the information, preferably well before that decision has to be made

◆ The midwife listening to the mother, never dismissing her concerns or questions, and being prepared to accept her decisions

◆ The woman feeling that she is making the decisions, that she will be supported in her decisions, able to assert her needs and accept responsibility for the consequences of her decisions

◆ The midwife providing safe, competent practice with effective communication and honesty throughout, where professional autonomy has also been respected

efficient records for pregnancy, labour and the postnatal period cannot be overemphasized. This is especially true if the woman is to see more than one midwife to facilitate continuity. If any disagreement arises afterwards, midwives' recordings of events may prove invaluable in explaining incidents or misunderstandings, when they may be called to account for actions or in actions in their practice. Symon (1997a) states that memory recall can be seriously affected by the passage of time and other significant events such as pain, effects of certain analgesics and retrospective knowledge. Consequently, the midwife has a responsibility to ensure that all records are accurate and consistent, providing a detailed history of the events as they take place. Retrospective knowledge may also unconsciously affect midwives' ability to record details, hence the need for contemporaneous records.

Accountability

The Midwives Rules and Code of Practice (UKCC 1998) and the Guidelines for Professional Practice (UKCC 1996) clearly state that every midwife is accountable for her own practice, which means that not only should they fully understand what they are doing, but also know why such actions are appropriate and safe. This obligates the midwife to keep up with current practice, critically evaluating research and using all the evidence available in an objective, effective and safe environment, providing opportunities for the best possible childbirth experiences.

Midwives are accountable for all practice issues (Dimond 1994a) (including any errors or misconduct) to:

◆ the mother and fetus/baby via the civil courts
◆ society via the criminal courts
◆ UKCC via the Professional Conduct Committee
◆ employers via the contract of employment.

Accountability to mother and fetus/baby

The midwife has a duty of care towards the mother and baby. This duty relates to care, treatments, information giving and record keeping. It also includes managing particular situations, including supervision and delegation of staff: 'all actions necessary to ensure that the mother and baby are safe' (Dimond 1994a: p 115). If the midwife fails to comply with this duty of care, with acceptable standards of practice, then the mother or baby may have recourse to sue for negligence in the civil courts.

In order to obtain compensation for an action of negligence (Dimond 1994a) the woman (or someone acting for her or/and the baby) would have to prove that:

1. The midwife owed a duty of care to the woman. This is usually easy to prove, especially if the midwife has previously been involved in the case or is employed by an authority who takes responsibility for service provision. Brazier (1992) reminds readers that the law on negligence does not oblige anyone to be a Good Samaritan, therefore if midwives observe a stranger in need of midwifery assistance, they are not legally obliged to help. However, they may feel morally obliged to lend assistance and once they do offer, they will then be deemed to have a duty of care towards that woman.

2. The midwife was in breach of that duty. In legal terms a satisfactory standard of care is determined by an appropriate representative body, who would determine what is considered a *reasonable* standard of care in any particular circumstance. (Brazier (1992) and Dimond (1994a) provide further discussion on how this is determined by the courts).

3. The harm (recognized by the courts as deserving compensation) was reasonably foreseeable. In other words, that not only was the midwife practising below an acceptable standard, but that the consequences (short and long term) of the actions, or non-actions, in question, could have been predicted as possibly harmful. Symon (1997b) reminds readers that the maintenance of a good standard of care and thorough record keeping cannot prevent allegations of negligence; however they should preclude a finding of negligence.

Accountability to society

The midwife, like all citizens, is accountable to society via the criminal courts. In relation to midwifery matters this may involve relevant acts of parliament. For example, those which govern the administration of medication, and the Midwives Rules (UKCC 1998) which have statutory force. For example, a midwife accused of theft (e.g. unexplained discrepancy in controlled drugs) may have to account for her actions in the criminal court (Dimond 1990).

Accountability to the UKCC

The UKCC is the elected statutory body for nurses, midwives and health visitors. They are responsible for setting the standards required for practice. If a member is accused of misconduct (e.g. breach of duty of care, misuse of drugs, practice outside their recognized sphere of practice), the Preliminary Proceedings Committee investigate such allegations and take appropriate action. This may involve referral to the Professional Conduct Committee, who may take action ranging from 'no further action', to suspension, or removal from the register following appropriate hearings (Jenkins 1995). Allegations may be submitted from a variety of sources including colleagues, supervisors of midwives, managers and the public. They are also automatically informed by the police or courts if a midwife is found guilty of a criminal offence (Jenkins 1995).

Accountability to the employer

Midwives who are employed are accountable to their employer as part of their contract. All policies/protocols applied by the employer must be followed, and generally that does not cause a problem as the midwife agrees and signs the employment contract. However, the employer may instigate protocols which may affect the midwife's practice and so midwives have a responsibility to ensure appropriate participation on committees who have authority for such decisions. The need for this collaboration was illustrated in 1994, in East Herts NHS Trust, when two midwives attended a woman labouring and giving birth in a birthing pool in her own home. The Trust had a protocol which *allowed* women to labour in water but not to give birth in water (Lewison 1996). The woman informed the midwives of her intention to use a birthing pool at home for pain relief and possibly for birth – she wanted to keep her options open. The midwives, recognizing their duty to care and the need to acquaint themselves with training and knowledge, appeared to have made every possible attempt to do so, and after assessing the then limited evidence available on waterbirth agreed to attend the woman. Their subsequent suspension from practice, followed by written warnings, raised many concerns nationally, not least the issues of women's right to choice, midwives autonomy to practice versus employer protocol. Lewison (1996) provides extensive discussion regarding this particular case but the issue for current discussion is how to avoid such situations in the future. Ideally, midwives and mothers should be well represented on protocol groups within their practice environment and such protocols should be supported by sound evidence.

Midwives may find a protocol imposed that causes concern, for example whereby it may be morally difficult for some midwives to support, or there may be some concerns that it is inadequate, unsafe or an erosion of women's right of choice. Midwives then have a responsibility to themselves and the women who may utilize the service, to investigate their concerns and make objective representation to their supervisor of midwives and manager. Such situations are always more effective if supported by a representative body, rather than individuals.

New therapies and strategies for relief of pain

It is important to note that not all strategies for the relief of pain involve pharmacological preparations and many complementary and/or alternative therapies are advocated nowadays. Midwives should maintain awareness of new ideas and strategies for pain relief. Although they may not be in a position to administer or directly provide new options, they should be conversant with advantages and disadvantages, including possible benefits and risks, in order to provide informed choices. With regard to new strategies, the Midwives Rules and Code (Rule 40 (2), 41 (1): UKCC 1998) are quite clear about midwives' responsibilities regarding acquiring adequate training in the acquisition of new skills.

This is further clarified in the Midwife's Code of Practice (No 20–23: UKCC 1994), which encourages consultation with the supervisor of midwives on such matters. Dimond (1995a) provides discussion on the potential 'legal minefield' midwives may face if they have training in complementary therapies which they may wish to use in midwifery practice. The Midwife's Code of Practice emphasizes the need for competence, as well as maternal consent and accountability. The stumbling block would appear to be the issues of competence and how this is defined. This is particularly problematic with therapies which are not widely used with women in labour. Their limited use may result in insufficient evidence of their benefits or risks. Again recourse to the supervisor of midwives may be invaluable if midwives wish to pursue non-orthodox spheres of practice, which if successful may further widen the choices available to women.

The other issue which Dimond (1995b) raises is that of when the mother may wish to use something that the midwife has no, or limited knowledge of (Reflective scenario 6.2). The increasing interest in complementary therapies may be related to women's dissatisfaction with available methods and a need

Reflective scenario 6.2

Katherine is 38 years old and expecting her first child. She has recently moved to the area and her antenatal care was conducted by her general practitioner where she used to live. The letter of transfer has limited information and suggests that pregnancy was uneventful. She has admitted herself in labour and when pain relief is discussed, she informs the midwife that her partner, Jacob, who is a herbalist, has prepared a mixture of herbs and other unidentified ingredients, which she is going to self administer throughout the labour. When questioned by the midwife, Jacob refuses to divulge the contents of his preparation. He is unaware if such a preparation has been used previously on a labouring woman but feels confident that it will not cause any harm to either mother or fetus – after all he would not put either in danger.

What should the midwife do in this situation?

to find more acceptable and suitable techniques. Midwives cannot delegate their responsibilities because of lack of knowledge and should make every attempt to investigate the risks and benefits, with any available evidence to understand the therapy, taking account of the fetus as well as the mother. Liaison with experts and the woman may also facilitate better understanding, however the midwife must always be concerned with safety and appropriateness. It may also be appropriate for the midwife to consider training, as part of widening the scope of practice. In the case of widely used therapies such as waterbirth it may be advisable to have written protocols and support groups to ensure adequate discussions on all available evidence and make sound judgements about agreed safe and effective practices.

ADMINISTRATION OF MEDICATION

The possession and administration of medication by midwives is controlled by the Medicine Act 1968, The Misuse of Drugs Act 1971, the Medicines Order 1983, the Misuse of Drugs Regulations 1985 and Medicinal Products: Prescriptions by Nurses etc. Act 1992 (Jones & Morris 1992). This is further regulated by Rule 41 of the Midwives Rules (UKCC 1998), which confirms the necessity for every midwife to be properly trained (either before or after initial registration) before becoming involved in the possession and administration of any medicine, including all analgesics.

The Midwives Code of Practice (UKCC 1998) expands on the details of individual responsibility in Paragraphs 15–19, which every midwife has a duty to be fully conversant with. Paragraphs 20–25 focus on prescription only and other medicines (which also includes herbal and homoeopathic medicines).

The prescription only drugs currently used are normally identified in local Standing Orders, which are drawn up by the consultant obstetrician, in agreement with the senior midwife/midwives. The obstetrician takes responsibility for the drugs authorized, however the midwives are always accountable for the drugs they administer, and should be fully aware of all the issues related to that particular drug. This is especially important with Standing Order drugs, because midwives exercise their judgement as to the appropriateness of administration without direct consultation with a medical practitioner (Simpson & Smith 1995).

Medication authorized in the Medicines Act (1968) may also be identified by local policies involving senior midwives, without consultation, which may be important for midwifery led care. Independent midwives need to discuss and agree individual lists with their supervisor of midwives (Simpson & Smith 1995). In 1997 the UKCC announced its intentions to pursue initiatives for midwives to prescribe some identified medication as part of their scope of practice, on the basis that simplifying the law is in line with the philosophy of women centred practices (UKCC 1997).

As with all areas of practice, the onus is with individual midwives to maintain accurate and current knowledge and understanding of all aspects of drugs (Banister 1997). If a midwife has concerns about a particular prescription, scrutiny via the British National Formulary, pharmaceutical company libraries or other appropriate resources should be sought, before administration or participation in administration of any medication. Midwives are accountable for all actions, even if directed by another professional.

CONCLUSION

Effective communication is the key to providing satisfactory care, which should support appropriate childbirth experiences for women. This is particularly true when contemplating the issues surrounding the woman's management of pain and discomfort in labour, and maintaining the midwife's professional integrity.

In order to facilitate the woman's autonomous decisions about her care, the midwife needs to understand and accept that the concept of respect for autonomy means enabling the woman to make the informed choices and supporting those rational choices without coercion, as well as accepting that the woman who made those choices has to take responsibility for them.

The midwife has a duty of care to inform and support women of the options available for pain relief. The information given should include benefits, risks and alternatives, which should be based on all the sound evidence available. It should also be given in a mode that the women can easily access and understand, providing sufficient time for her to reflect on the information and question its appropriateness for her – ideally during the antenatal period. This exercise should be achieved in such a way as to enable the woman to make fully informed decisions about the preferred choices for her. Women who give birth in hospital may feel intimidated by the foreign and often hostile looking surroundings and may need the midwife to act as advocate for them, which involves knowing individual needs and expectations, and being prepared to support autonomous decisions.

Midwives cannot lose sight of the fact that they have to practise within their defined scope of practice, which is governed by legal as well as moral frameworks, in an attempt to meet women's needs and expectations. They also need to constantly strive to ensure that all practice is up to date and evidence based, being mindful not to undertake any practices which they have not been adequately prepared for or feel competent in. They should also utilize the resources available to them to support practice, such as the supervisor of midwives and further education opportunities on women's needs and new techniques for relief of pain.

Effective communication is an essential element in avoiding conflict, which may also involve appropriate multidisciplinary liaison and support. This includes encouraging midwives' and mothers' active participation in planning service provision, including development of protocols which may influence practice. This can only lead to a maintenance of satisfactory standards and a service which provides choice in meeting individual women's needs.

At the end of an encounter the midwife should be able to evaluate the service provided as effective and safe, having accommodated the woman with the best possible experience for her particular birthing challenge.

ANNOTATED BIBLIOGRAPHY

Dimond B 1994 Legal aspects of midwifery. Books for Midwives, Cheshire

Legal issues in midwifery practice may often cause concern for practitioners, and this book by the well-known author Bridgit Dimond provides a comprehensive guide to many of the legal concerns practitioners may have. It is easy to read, and outlines the basic framework of the legal system that is specific to being a registered midwife, before moving on to the more complex issues which midwives need to be aware of. It is a useful reference for experienced practitioners and provides a general guide to the legal framework for student midwives and new practitioners. Relevant legal cases provide a useful model for discussion on various situations and each chapter ends with some pertinent questions which can inform valid discussion for all who practise midwifery and related health care positions.

Dickson A 1992 A woman in your own right: assertiveness and you. Quartet Books, London

Anne Dickson's book describes assertiveness as the art of clear, honest, direct communication. It provides an interesting read for all women who would wish to question or control their own lives, in particular in relation to becoming more assertive. It considers the concepts of self worth and confidence in knowing and governing one's life in a way that can empower women to make informed choices and enjoy the security of knowing those choices were right for them at that time. It is a recommended read for midwives and women – pregnant or not – as it could change the reader's life for ever, by making some women more aware of the skills and power of assertiveness.

Frith L 1996 Ethics and midwifery: issues in contemporary practice. Butterworth Heinemann, London

Moral decision making is an essential element to good midwifery practices, and it is important for midwives to be fully informed of the contemporary issues which they may face in their practice today, as well as considering how practice may need to change to meet the needs and expectations of women. This book, edited by Lucy Frith, provides well-written, extensive chapters on some of the diverse ethical issues which midwives and health care professionals may face today. It looks at choice and control of childbirth, as well as focusing on technological and professional issues. It is well referenced and the variety of author styles add to the value of this book.

REFERENCES

Banister C 1997 The midwife's pharmacopeia. Books for Midwives Press, Cheshire
Beauchamp TL, Childress JF 1994 Principles of biomedical ethics, 4th edn. Oxford University Press, Oxford
Brazier M 1992 Medicine, patients and the law. Penguin Books, London
Department of Health 1993 Changing Childbirth Report to the Expert Maternity Group. HMSO, London
Dickson A 1992 A woman in your own right: assertiveness and you. Quartet Books, London
Dimond B 1990 Legal aspects of nursing. Prentice Hall, London
Dimond B 1994a Legal aspects of midwifery. Books for Midwives Press, Cheshire
Dimond B 1994b The midwife's power to prescribe. Modern Midwife Nov: 34
Dimond B 1995a Complementary therapy and the midwife. Modern Midwife Feb: 32
Dimond B 1995b Complementary therapy and the mother's wishes. Modern Midwife Mar: 34
Gillon R 1985 Philosophical medical ethics. John Wiley, Chichester
International Confederation of Midwives (ICM) 1994 An International Code of Ethics for Midwives. Nursing Ethics 1(1)
Jenkins R 1995 The law and the midwife. Blackwell Science, Oxford
Jones MA, Morris AE 1992 Blackstone's statutes on medical law. Blackstone's, London
Jones S 1994 Ethics in midwifery. Mosby-Year Book Europe, London
Lewison H 1996 Choices in childbirth: areas of conflict. In: Frith L (ed) Ethics and midwifery: issues in contemporary practice. Butterworth Heinemann, London, ch 2, pp 36–50
Mander R 1993 Who chooses the choices? Modern Midwife 3: 23–25
Mander R 1996 Failure to deliver: ethical issues relating to epidural analgesia in uncomplicated labour. In: Frith L (ed) Ethics and midwifery: issues in contemporary practice. Butterworth Heinemann, Oxford, ch 3, pp 52–71
Sandell J 1997 Midwives burnout and continuity of care. British Journal of Midwifery 5(2): 106–111
Schott J 1994 The importance of encouraging women to think for themselves. British Journal of Midwifery 2(1): 3–4
Simpson D, Smith R 1995 Drugs, the law and the midwife: 1. British Journal of Midwifery 3(8): 420–422
Symon A 1997a Midwives and litigation: allegations of clinical error. British Journal of Midwifery 5(1): 17–20
Symon A 1997b Recollections of patients: versions of the truth. British Journal of Midwifery 5(6): 327–329
UKCC 1994 The midwife's code of practice. UKCC, London
UKCC 1996 Guidelines for professional practice. UKCC, London
UKCC 1997 No 20 Summer 1997 Register. UKCC, London
UKCC 1998 Midwives rules and code of practice. UKCC, London

7

Alternative therapies for pain relief

Christine Grabowska

KEY ISSUES

- Giving information
- Women in control
- Being in 'tune', midwife with woman
- Touch
- Massage
- Therapeutic touch
- Guided imagery – relaxation
- Hypnosis
- Water to aid birth
- Complementary therapies

INTRODUCTION

Pain in labour is an essential warning system, as it brings about the dramatic changes which warn woman that she is entering motherhood. This chapter discusses how women may be supported through the painful process of labour by natural methods of pain-coping mechanisms, which may help women to go with what is happening to their bodies.

GIVING INFORMATION

Women want information about how to cope with the pain of labour; unfortunately, many women set their sights on labour, and look no further. It is as if they will automatically know how to nurture once the labour is over, if this is the case then they, by implication, will know how to labour also without instruction. However, women are often driven by fear – you can hear them saying 'give me an anaesthetic', 'knock me out', 'wake me up when it's over'. The information that is often received from professionals reinforces women's fear because they are told how it will be possible to escape the pain (Leap 1992, Hunt & Symonds 1995), and hence to be passively involved in birthing of their babies.

Culturally pain is seen as bad and therefore needs to be abolished (Bendelow 1993). Should we, for instance, abolish fetal screening to avoid bad news (Brand & Yancey 1995)? Some women have been socialized to shun the pain of labour, while other women have been shown ways of coping with it (Jeffery et al 1989, Helman 1990, Vincent Priya 1992, Jordan 1993, Bendelow & Williams 1995). We live in a country that uses technology for industry, factories, offices and the land. It follows therefore that we should use our 'advancement' for childbirth. Technology has convinced us that our lives can be made easier by the use of its products – like the washing machine, the lift, the motor car – so why not childbirth (Wagner 1986, Davies 1996)? We are talking about people here and not machines – that's the difference!

WOMEN IN CONTROL

The pain is not the whole picture. The woman has a mind, emotions and feelings that stretch well beyond the physiological process of giving birth (Morse & Park 1988). She is an integral part of the body that will give birth to the baby. She can control her hormonal response depending on whether she wants to labour now, tomorrow or the next day. She can control whether it is 'safe' – and may switch her labour off (through the catecholamine response) at the command of her brain (commonly seen when she arrives on the labour ward or when strangers come into the labour room; Jowitt 1993). She will decide when to push her baby out. If you ask women, they often have no conscious awareness of the way they were in tune with and therefore in control of their birth process.

BEING IN 'TUNE', MIDWIFE WITH WOMAN

Women are amazing! We will explore the possibilities for the midwife to be 'with them' in the birth process, and support their body's ability to produce its analgesia – commonly known as endorphins. Encouragement of the fear process will switch off or prevent the release of these chemicals. The environment and people have to be adjusted to each individual woman's fine attunement, rather than an expectation that the woman should fit in with the environment of the labour ward; which has its standard prescriptions available for pain relief, while the attendants are unable to reduce her fear (Hunt & Symonds 1995).

We know that in order for the physiological process to have the best chance of working we need to consider reducing the outside stimuli (Newton et al 1966, Kitzinger 1988). Some of the ways of achieving this are – dimming the lights, 'allowing' a place for the woman to hide (this has usually been the toilet and bathroom). 'Allowing' the woman to close her eyes, while the attendants have a distant presence and whisper when they share the same room. This helps to create a 'safe' environment for the woman so that she can relax and trust her labour process. In addition she needs to trust her attendants to be her strong advocates. So what qualities does the advocate need?

First, to be able to put routine practices and procedures to the side and listen to the woman. Second, to be able to support the environment. Third, to be the gatekeeper – that is, preventing others from coming to have a look. Finally, among other things, attendants need to have the unfaltering belief in the woman's ability to labour and give birth to her baby (Sakala 1988).

Once women trust the environment and their attendants, thus relaxing into the process of labour, they can 'switch off'. A woman who is labouring at home will be familiar and relaxed in her environment. You will observe how she changes position frequently, how she moves her pelvis spontaneously to aid descent of the fetus. She moves to aid fetal position in her pelvis and how she never chooses to lay flat on her back (Parsons 1994, Simkin 1995)! She will choose positions to relieve the pain of labour. She may also moan and groan – a way of relieving the pent-up tension and thus reduce her awareness of the pain. The midwife will watch over this process, knowing what a privilege it is to be the onlooker – to know the woman trusts her attendant so much that she is able to give way to the unique way that her body will unfold.

The woman usually gets to the point in her labour when she has had enough, wants to go home, even though she is here already, and considers an epidural. The midwife recognizes this and now needs to use all her resources to help this woman work through this stage because very soon this woman will give birth to her baby (Scarry 1985, Fordham & Dunn 1994, Niven 1994).

The midwife will whisper words of encouragement, but the woman may scream and possibly swear back. The midwife may suggest different positions, hip swaying, she may get hot towels for the woman's back (but once you begin this she will want a continuous stream of hot towels until the birth). This may be the time to suggest a shower or a bath (Brown 1982). The sound of running water is important. Still water, in the bath, will have the effect of relaxing the labour while running water indicates the flowing, continuous process – so keep the taps running in a bath (Sakala 1988).

Some women appreciate your close presence at this time. You must be calm and totally centred yourself (Sakala 1988) – clear your mind of all of your own life's issues and be wholly with this woman – this ensures that she will not be aware of any negative feelings. Women in labour seem to have a heightened intuition, so she will feel the way you feel about her! Transmit the way you care about her, think she is fantastic, positively appreciate her strength, wish her an easy and uncomplicated labour and believe in her ability to do this. As you send her positive thoughts – watch her melt, her shoulders will drop and the contractions take a break, so that she regains her strength and resources for the second stage of labour.

Negative thoughts, words or deeds in most cases will create the self-fulfilling prophecy. How many times have you seen the comment 'She will have a caesarean' become reality (Sakala 1988)? Be aware of where your loyalties lie (with woman, with institution, with doctor or elsewhere) and then you will know whether you are acting as a midwife, administrator or nurse. A midwife can truly support the birth process (Rich 1977, Wagner 1986), and this can be aided with complementary therapies.

TOUCH

Some women may want to be touched (Montagu 1978, Feltham 1991) – remember that you will continue to transmit the same emotions through touch (Simkin 1995). Therefore you do not have to say anything. If she wants a massage – massage slowly because you can show anxiety when you rub fast. Do not touch her spine because you have not been trained in the same way as an osteopath or chiropractor, and any pressure may lead to manipulation of the joints. This is because of the effects of progesterone on all smooth muscle and ligaments.

MASSAGE

Massage can be done over clothes or with direct skin contact. The woman may have bought some aromatherapy oils of her choice to use especially for massage. If she is using relaxing oils you will feel the effect too (Reed & Norfolk 1993).

Using the whole of your hand and using long firm strokes start from the shoulders, move down the back, buttocks and to the legs (vary the strokes on her legs from the front to the back). You will help to relieve muscle tension while producing the profound psychological stimulation that can create the thought, in the woman, of moving the baby downwards, opening her up while she is relaxing.

A woman may not want massage but may wish to have manual pressure applied to her sacrum for pain relief (Sakala 1988, Simkin 1995). Put the heel of your hand over her sacrum and the other hand on top of the first, bend your knees – now let your weight flow into her back. You could try outward movements of your hands from the sacroiliac joints to the wings of the ileum, the strong message is of opening the pelvis. Be guided by what she finds feels beneficial. If she has calm attendants (partner or friends) they could be shown these techniques, so that you can be freed up when she starts to grunt and breath hold. Often attendants take their cues from the midwife – so if the midwife panics so does everyone else. If the midwife laughs and talks loudly – so does everyone else. The midwife is crucial in protecting the calm and peace of the birthing environment.

THERAPEUTIC TOUCH

Pain sensations and touch travel along the same nerve fibres (Doehring 1989) (see Ch. 3). Midwives are good at massaging backs in labour and have watched women relax and their levels of anxiety decrease as a result of touching. Touching is a way of letting people know you care about, accept and support them. However, if touching is performed in a rushed, rough manner with quick movements, this may be perceived as frustration, anger or impatience on the practitioner's part. The meaning attached to this may be that the touch is uncaring and cold (Wright 1995). Rubin (1963) showed that mothers who had received meaningful touch during labour, handled their babies more effectively than mothers who were treated impersonally and remotely during labour.

Some people, it must be remembered, do not like to be touched. Wright (1995) tells us that generally it is safe to assess this by looking at the reaction to a handshake (which is an acceptable form of touching, in this culture). Body tensing or facial grimacing will alert the midwife to the woman's distress. Equally, if the woman releases the midwife's hand quickly this is an indication that touch may not be acceptable. On the other hand, if the woman allows her hand to remain, or clings to the midwife's hand, she may be comfortable with touch. However, this is not conclusive. It is best to test this further, through the performance of routine tasks. What happens if you use a flannel gently on her forehead, or hold her hand while you talk? If she is accepting of touch, then you may offer a massage. Massage can release emotions and 'baggage', as well as reducing nervous tension, this alone will help the muscles to relax. It will increase the circulation to the skin, but at the same time, decrease the heart rate and blood pressure (Feltham 1991). Therapeutic touch (TT), on the other hand, does not require touch, but the woman must be happy to allow the practitioner to move their hands over her body at a distance of about 4–6 inches. (10–15 cm). Feltham (1991) says that TT reduces the length of labour, and delivery complications.

TT does not involve the need for touching. It is a system of therapy that has evolved from the USA and Canada, where it is taught in over 80 universities and hospitals. It was formally recognized in 1990, by the College of Nurses of Ontario through implementation into their 'Standards of Practice'. TT is also endorsed by the National League for Nursing in the USA. It has become part of the nurses' curriculum. There are purported to be no side-effects, it is inexpensive, does not need technology or other space-occupying equipment to be performed. It can be used without a doctor's order; even though training is recommended, there is no requirement for certification to practice.

TT works on the premise that there is a human energy electromagnetic field that is imperceptible to the human eye, it surrounds a person's body. Martha Rogers (1980) believes that humans are the energy fields. This field can be photographed by Kirlian photography. Some people would describe the energy field as an aura, and others would say that it is the equivalent to what the traditional Chinese therapists refer to as 'qi'. The aura is described as different layers to include the physical body, the etheric body, the astral body, the mental body and the causal body. This energy is said to be in direct contact with environmental energy. These two energies flow together and are interchangeable. The qi, on the other hand, is said to flow in a system of channels (or meridians) throughout the body. Therapies such as acupuncture or Shiatsu are said to manipulate or change the flow of energy. Again these channels are not seen by the naked eye, even at post-mortem (Figure 7.1).

TT was recorded in the 1960s by a biochemist (Grad 1961, 1963). He used a healer, Oskar Estebany, to conduct his experiments. But it was a nurse, Dolores Krieger, who brought TT into nurse education establishments. She worked with a healer, Dora Kunz, who became her mentor. They believed that the theoretical basis for this phenomenon came from the Indian/Ayurvedic beliefs in prana (another term for qi). It is perhaps more commonly known that prana is the energy force that is referred to during the practice of yoga. Miller (1979), Jurgens et al (1987), Turton (1989), Leduc (1989), Bolstad (1990), Harrison (1990) and Thayer (1990) explained the meaning of TT and how it developed in the field of nursing.

The human energy field theory has many promoters expounding its benefits, however this is mainly anecdotal (MacRae 1979, Bulbrook 1984, Newshaw 1989, Payne 1989). There are thought to be over two dozen doctoral dissertations, dozens of master theses and many other studies on TT that have been funded by the National Institute of Health. There is even less work available around the area of human pregnancy and birth. The literature refers to Albert Einstein's work on the theory of relativity (1905). It is thought that physics is the area of science that proves this energy field (Chopra 1989).

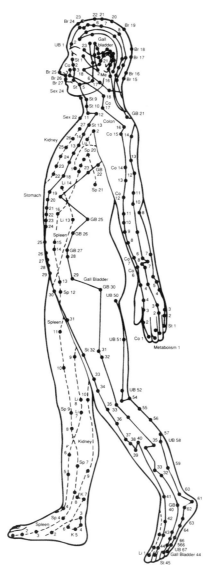

Figure 7.1 Illustration of acupuncture channels and points. A representation of where the qi flows through the channels. (Reproduced with permission from Tiran & Mack 1995.)

The work that has been carried out includes that of Grad (1961), who showed that the wounds of mice healed faster, and again in 1964 he showed how plants grew faster when worked on by a healer. Krieger (1972, 1974) showed that haemoglobin levels can be raised by the use of TT. Quinn (1982) followed up Heidt's (1981) study and showed that the response from the patient did not change if physical touch or 'hands off' TT was used to reduce anxiety. Quinn (1989) also demonstrated that TT will decrease blood pressure. Heidt (1981) and Gagne (1994) recommended TT for reducing anxiety. Keller & Bzdek's (1986) and Meehan's (1985) work led them to recommend TT for the reduction of pain. Wirth (1990) and Wirth (1993), in their study of wound healing, resulted in TT speeding up the process of healing. Reduction of stress was shown to be another adage to TT by the work of Kramer (1990) and Olson et al (1992).

The critics (Glickman & Burns 1996) have denigrated the use of public money to discover the efficaciousness of TT, and referred to the Rosa (1998) study. This study was conducted by a 9-year-old for her school science project! The results showed that practitioners could only discover the human energy field by chance. The article concluded that all professional use of TT should be abandoned. Whatever its methods, the outcomes seem to be the proof! Even if the placebo effect could be 'blamed', a Channel 4 programme asking if some treatments worked by magic backed up its efficaciousness (Buckman & Sabbagh 1993).

TT involves re-balancing either excess or deficient energy, similar to the Chinese theories of Yin and Yang. Yin refers to the deeper, more internal pathways and organs, while Yang refers to the more superficial pathways and the hollow organs. Illness or pain will block the energy field! The practitioner has to remove these energy blockages in order to alleviate the pain, as well as have an effect on the mental and emotional well being of the woman. There are five practices to be followed for TT to be successful:

◆ centring
◆ assessment
◆ clearing
◆ intervention
◆ evaluation.

Centring is used to achieve a calm, meditative state. Some people refer to this as grounding. However, unless well practised, this can be hard to achieve in the daily hustle and bustle of a ward. Clearly, calmness should be the atmosphere of a labour ward, so that the woman can relax, and consequently the practitioner can 'switch off'. The practitioner should remain alert and may use meditative or visualization practices to centre themselves. At this stage the practitioner has to believe that energy will follow thought (Simington 1993). TT has as its basis unconditional love and compassion, so the practitioner makes a mental affirmation to help the woman. McClelland (Borysenko 1985) suggests that these feelings in the practitioner will improve the immune response.

Assessment of the body is carried out by moving the hands (palms down) over the clothed body in order to feel areas of imbalance. This is very subtle. The practitioner is 'quiet' and 'listens', it is an intuitive process. The sensation felt through the hands can be a tingling, heat/cold, or a heaviness or it may be a 'drawing' feeling.

Clearing is done by a sweeping downward movement of the hands. Although practitioners do this differently, the idea is that they are removing the energy blockages. The hands will concentrate on the areas where an imbalance was felt. It is at this point that the woman will feel relaxation and the pain will tend to ease. TT is thought to affect the autonomic nervous system by decreasing the sympathetic response (Mackey 1995). It is thought that, at this stage, when the woman is deeply relaxed, a state of self healing takes place (Sayre-Adams 1994). Mackey (1995) believes that not only is there a reduction in the amount of pain felt, but the period of pain relief will extend well beyond the period that TT is being performed.

The intervention phase is where the practitioner actively sends energy, through her hands, to the areas of deficit. If a cool area has previously been felt, then the practitioner will aim to warm this area. This could be away from the area of pain. The idea here is to make the energy field smooth, uniform and flowing.

Finally, evaluation is completed by making a judgement to determine whether the rebalancing is complete. The practitioner must now 'close down', by mentally removing themselves from the woman and allowing the woman to rest peacefully, with little disruption. The whole TT can last up to an hour. However, the average treatment times are about 15–20 minutes. Mackey (1995) says that TT has an effect on the practitioner too. The practitioner becomes more self aware, may decide to change their own lifestyle and be more appreciative of their surroundings.

GUIDED IMAGERY – RELAXATION

Guided imagery can be used to change attitudes and develop self awareness. It is a simple technique using relaxation to heighten the senses. The ideal place to introduce this is in the antenatal period, so that it can be used for labour. Having talked a woman through a relaxation sequence (Sutcliffe 1991), a scenario is usually presented but the relaxed person has to develop the scenario in their own mind. This technique is often used in stress management courses. It usually involves imagining areas such as a wood, and walking through the trees; the sea or a beach; a river or a refreshing walk through hills and so on. The scenario will depend on where the woman will choose to be her 'safe haven'.

An example of one such imagery (but you could develop many more) is give in Box 7.1.

When women feel panicky in labour it is simple enough to let them use their imagination, through the prepared guided imagery.

> **Box 7.1** An example of guided imagery
>
> *To be read slowly and softly in a calm voice, with many pauses, following a relaxation*
>
> Imagine you are in the house of your dreams ... go to your favourite room ... how big is it ... how many windows has it got ... what do they look like ... look out of one of the windows ... what do you see ... is it day or night ... are there other buildings ... is it green ... is there a garden ... what's outside ... what colour is the sky ... can you see the sun or the moon and stars ... can you see any animals ... what's the weather like ... come back into the room look at the ceiling – its colour, its shape and if there's anything special about it ... look at the walls, what is it you really like about them ... is there anything on the walls ... look at the floor, what are you standing on ... is it the same all over the floor ... what furniture do you have ... is there any electrical equipment ... are there any plants ... has it got a fireplace, what does it look like ... can you smell anything ... go and touch something that you like the feel of ... can you hear anything ... what is it about this room that makes you feel so good ... is there anyone with you in this room ... what are you doing, saying and feeling ... what do you enjoy about the person you have with you ... now remember you can come into this room at any time, it is your special place to enjoy and feel pleasure.

Preparation can be very simple! Introduce the notion of the stresses in everyone's life, perhaps in an antenatal group. The group may volunteer examples; and in the same way ask the group for their solutions to decrease the amount of stress that they feel. You can suggest the use of relaxation using imagery and ask the group if they would like to try it. A positive response is usual. The effect of this preparation is that the group are now more receptive to trying it out.

Once you have worked through the relaxation and the guided imagery the group can choose to discuss it or take it home with them to think about. At the next group meeting you might ask them if they have been back to this room and see if they will reveal their feeling about it and start talking about using it for relaxation and gaining a feeling of safety during labour. Once they have grown comfortable using this imagery, you only need to suggest it during labour rather than read the whole thing again.

HYPNOSIS

The first recorded use of hypnosis for analgesia was for a tooth extraction in 1821, but by 1823 it was noted that it was used for labour (LeCron 1971).

Some women may have attended a self-hypnosis workshop during the antenatal period (Boot 1987, Lawless 1992, Jenkins & Pritchard 1993, Arthurs 1994). This is usually carried out in groups of four. Women learn to relax first by themselves – without falling asleep – and then using their imagination, turn off the reception of pain by the brain. They will usually be given a word that is repeated about three times along with a body movement that has to be performed simultaneously (this is to prevent going into a hypnotic state because they hear the word by accident).

The midwife can assist the woman who wishes to use self-hypnosis by protecting the environment as already discussed. The woman will remove herself from this state easily by strangers walking in the room, by loud noises, by people holding everyday conversations around her, by being touched without warning or permission (Vadurro & Butts 1982). She has got to trust the environment. Self-hypnosis is a method that the woman controls but its effectiveness depends on the midwife. This will work on a labour ward where the woman and her choices are respected. Wine (1988), Jenkins & Pritchard (1993) and Harmon et al (1990) all show the positive effects of using hypnosis to reduce the need for other forms of pain relief during labour – no undesirable effects were noted.

WATER TO AID BIRTH

Waterbirth is not 'new'. The first record of waterbirth showed that it took place in France in 1803 (Church 1989). In the 1960s Tjarkovsky brought waterbirths to the forefront exploring the benefits for the baby (Sidenbladh 1983). Odent (1984) came across waterbirths by accident (when a woman did not want to get out of the water for the birth). The Winterton Report (House of Commons Health Committee 1992) recommended that women should be provided with 'the option of a birthing pool where this is practicable'. The first birthing pool was installed in this country in 1987 and 89% of NHS provider units in England and Wales have at some time made provision for waterbirth (Alderice 1995b).

Immersion in water is well known for reducing anxiety (Levine 1984), increasing the release of natural opiates (Milner 1983), while reducing catecholamine secretion (Odent 1983) and ultimately giving pain relief (Simkin & Dickerson 1990). Movement is easier in water because of the feeling of weightlessness; women may thus feel more in control of their labour process (Jepson 1989, Balaskas & Gordon 1990, Garland 1995, Flint 1996).

Some of the issues that have led to the bad press over waterbirths need to be considered. The recommended water temperature should be between 35 and 37°C and the maternal temperature needs to be between 36.5°C and

37°C. If either is too hot this could lead to fetal tachycardia (Nightingale 1994), brain damage and possible death to the baby (Attwood & Lewis 1994). If the temperature is below this recommended limit then the baby may need treatment for hypothermia (Gallanan 1980).

McCandlish & Renfrew (1993) point out that there is no increased risk of infection by labouring and birthing in water. The associated approximate mortality has been reported as 1.24 per 1000 (Alderice 1995a) in water. To date there is no evidence to show that this practice should discontinue (Alderice 1995a).

COMPLEMENTARY THERAPIES

The British Medical Association (BMA) (1993) considered that there are about 160 possible complementary therapies. The midwife must have received training in their use (UKCC (United Kingdom Central Council for Nursing, Midwifery and Health Visiting), 1998). The 'Midwives Rules and Code of Practice' (UKCC 1998) provides guidance for practice. However, the majority of NHS trusts would want to see qualifications related to the therapy prior to their use. This means that usually the woman would have to invite a practitioner of the therapy of her choosing to be present (usually with the permission of the manager/consultant), or that she brings in whatever she wants to use and gives it to herself. This creates a moral dilemma for the midwife who, on the one hand, wishes to support the woman and, on the other, wishes to obey rules 40 and 41 (UKCC 1998). In order to fulfil this rule, it would be good practice to gain some knowledge of the therapy by gathering information about the method (Royal College of Midwives 1989). Many midwives, for instance, are already familiar with raspberry leaf tea, taken in the latter weeks of pregnancy to ensure an effective and efficient labour of shorter duration and with minimal pain. It is said to produce great tonifying effects on the uterus (Stapleton 1995). Some women may wish to continue drinking this throughout labour and the puerperium, ensuring a coordinated labour and an uneventful involution of the uterus (Sakala 1988). Midwives would benefit from finding more out about this herb before endorsing it!

There is no doubt that complementary therapies support midwives in their role of being with woman.

Some therapies rely heavily on the midwife's presence while others rely on her ability to use her knowledge of the remedies that will help the woman to stay in control of her labour. But all of them promote the midwife as a healer (Achterberg 1990).

CONCLUSION

Women need the confidence to believe in their own abilities prior to labour. The midwife, who has faith in women and their power, can inspire women to believe in themselves and thus reduce overall anxiety and need for pharmacological pain relief. Women are amazing in how they birth their babies. In the end it is the way the midwife supported the woman that becomes the reason that women say 'Thank you – you are amazing'.

Useful resources

◆ The General Council & Register of Consultant Herbalists, 32 King Edward Road, Swansea SA1 4LL, UK. Tel: +44 (0) 1792 655 886

◆ The Dr Edward Bach Centre, Mount Vernon, Sotwell, Wallingford, Oxon OX10 0PZ, UK. Tel: +44 (0) 1491 834 678

◆ British Wheel of Yoga, 1 Hamilton Place, Boston Road, Sleaford, Lincolnshire NG34 7ES, UK. Tel: +44 (0) 1529 306851

◆ Shirley Price Aromatherapy Training, 3 Latymer Close, Braybrooke, Market Harborough, Leicester LE16 8LN, UK. Tel: +44 (0) 1455 615466

◆ The Council for Acupuncture, 179 Gloucester Place, London NW1 6DX, UK. Tel: +44 (0) 171 724 5756

◆ The Society of Homoeopaths, 2 Artizan Road, Northampton NN1 4HU, UK. Tel: +44 (0) 1604 621400

◆ The Association of Reflexologists, 27 Old Gloucester Street, London WC1N 2XX, UK. Tel: +44 (0) 870 567 3320

◆ British Hypnotherapy Association, 1 Wythburn Place, London W1H 5WL, UK. Tel: +44 (0) 171 262 8852 and (0) 171 723 4443

◆ British Shiatsu Council, 121 Sheen Road, Richmond, Surrey TW9 1YJ, UK. Tel: +44 (0) 181 852 1080

◆ The Spiritualist Association of Great Britain, 33 Belgrave Square, London SW1X 8QB, UK. Tel: +44 (0) 171 2353351

ANNOTATED BIBLIOGRAPHY

Buenting JA 1993 Human energy fields and birth: implications for research and practice. Advanced Nursing Science 15(4): 53–59

This article recognizes that there is not a wealth of information surrounding therapeutic touch and labour in people, as opposed to animals. It tells us that it is a unique area where midwives can conduct research away from a biomedical model of childbirth. It describes what is meant by 'energy fields' and includes not just therapeutic touch but also meditation, visualization and imagery. It tells of the positive birth outcomes possible with the use of these techniques and urges midwives to gain skills in not just therapeutic touch but also acupressure/shiatsu, in order to provide a better service to women.

Cradle to Grave 1998 Debate on Alternatives to Modern Medicine. Video. Channel 4

This debate is around a table. The members of the panel include traditional as well as complementary practitioners, scientists and a journalist, who is also the editor of the journal 'What the doctors don't tell you'. It is interspersed with documentary evidence that adds to the debate. The debate includes: conversations on the environment; antibiotics; drug iatrogenesis; biotechnology; biomedicine. The question that seems to surround the debate is 'to whose advantage' or 'who will profit from traditional medicine'? It is a balanced debate that does not appear to get too heated and gives an insight into the wider issues that surround, for instance, choosing a method of pain relief.

Ernst E 1999 Complementary medicine: too good to be true? Journal of the Royal Society of Medicine V: 92: 1–2

This article discusses the issues of why people pay for complementary therapies when there is a free system of health care. It describes the potential clientele and the advantages of complementary medicine. The article questions how complementary medicine aligns itself with 'evidence based practice' and asks traditional practitioners not to be dismissive but to use databases and other resources in order to build up knowledge of complementary therapies.

Eslinger MR 1998 Hypnosis principles and applications: an adjunct to health care. Seminars in Perioperative Nursing 7(1): 39–45

This article extols the virtues of hypnosis as a complementary therapy based on its historical longevity. It explains what it is, what it does and what it can achieve. It is easy to read and gives an insight into the potential of hypnosis.

Hepworth S, Gaskell T, Bassett C 1996 Extended roles: a holistic approach to pain. Nursing Standard 10 (Jan): 18–20

This article is written by nurses who manage a pain clinic. They tell of the virtues of integrating the physical with the psyche, when working out treatment plans. They describe the procedures for dealing with patients, as well as mentioning the techniques they teach people to use at home.

Saks M (ed) 1992 Alternative medicine in Britain. Clarendon, Oxford

This book takes a look at alternative medicine historically and refers to homoeopathy, healing, osteopathy, herbalism, chiropractic and acupuncture. It looks at the relationship with traditional medicine and has two chapters (2 and 7) relating to pregnancy (one of these is by Ann Oakley – Chapter 2). These chapters discuss the association that has been made with midwives and witches and later the exclusion of women from a medical training. It acknowledges the respected status of women healers, historically, and how this has changed with the rise of medicine – it tells of the local midwife being ousted with the birth of legislation for registration of midwives. The political debate between traditional and complementary therapies is dealt with, and questions asked about the integration of complementary medicine under the medical umbrella. It also mentions the potential loss of profit to the big multinational companies and the debate that this engenders.

REFERENCES

Achterberg J 1990 Woman as healer. Shambala Publications
Alderice F 1995a Labour and birth in water in England and Wales. British Medical Journal 310: 837
Alderice F 1995b A national study of labour and birth in water. Midwives Jan: 3–11
Arthurs G 1994 Hypnosis and acupuncture in pregnancy. British Journal of Midwifery 2(10): 495–498
Attwood G, Lewis R 1994 Pool rules. Nursing Times 90(3): 72–73
Balaskas J, Gordon Y 1990 Waterbirth. Unwins, London
Bendelow G 1993 Pain perceptions, emotions and gender. Sociology of Health and Illness 15: 273–294
Bendelow G, Williams SJ 1995 Transcending the dualisms: towards a sociology of pain. Sociology of Health and Illness 17: 139–165
Bolstad R 1990 Healing through the human energy field. New Zealand Nursing Journal Jul: 21–22
Boot M 1987 Hypnosis in pregnancy, labour and the puerperium. Journal of the Association of Chartered Physiotherapists in Obstetrics and Gynaecology 60: 30–31
Borysenko J 1985 Healing motives: an interview with David C. McClelland. Advances 2(2): 29–41
Brand P, Yancey P 1995 Pain: the gift nobody wants. Marshall Pickering, London
British Medical Association 1993 Complementary medicine, new approaches to good practice. Oxford University Press, Oxford
Brown C 1982 Therapeutic effects of bathing during labour. Journal of Nurse-Midwifery 27: 13–16
Buckman R, Sabbagh K 1993 Magic or medicine: an investigation into healing. MacMillan, London
Bulbrook M 1984 Bulbrook's model of therapeutic touch. Canadian Nurse 80(11): 30–33
Chopra D 1989 Quantum healing. Bantam Books, New York
Church L 1989 Waterbirth: one birthing centre's observations. Journal of Nurse-Midwifery 34: 165–169
Davies S 1996 Divided loyalties: the problem of normality. British Journal of Midwifery 4(6): 285–286
Doehring KM 1989 Relieving pain through touch. Advances in Clinical Care 4(5): 32
Feltham E 1991 Therapeutic touch and massage. Nursing Standard 5(45): 26–28
Flint C 1996 Waterbirth and the role of the midwife. In: Beech BL (ed) Waterbirth unplugged. Books for Midwives Press, Hale, Cheshire, ch 10

Fordham M, Dunn V 1994 Alongside the person in pain: holistic care and nursing practice. Baillière Tindall, London

Gagne D 1994 The effects of therapeutic touch and relaxation therapy in reducing anxiety. Archives of Psychiatric Nursing 8(3): 184

Gallanan T 1980 Underwater birth. Mothering Summer: 59–61

Garland D 1995 Waterbirth: an attitude to care. Books for Midwives Press, Hale, Cheshire

Glickman R, Burns J 1996 If therapeutic touch works, prove it! RN – Medical Economics at Montvale, NJ 59(12): 76

Grad B 1961 An unorthodox method of treatment of wound healing in mice. International Journal of Parapsychology 3: 5–24

Grad B 1963 A telekinetic effect on plant growth. International Journal of Parapsychology 5: 117–133

Grad B 1964 A telekinetic effect on plant growth. International Journal of Parapsychology 6: 473–498

Harmon TM, Hynan MY, Tyre TE 1990 Improved obstetric outcomes using hypnotic analgesia. Consulting and Clinical Psychology 58: 525–530

Harrison MJ 1990 Therapeutic touch. New Zealand Nursing Journal May: 23–24

Heidt PR 1981 Effect of therapeutic touch on anxiety of hospitalised patients. Nursing Research 30(1): 32–37

Helman CG 1990 Culture, health and illness. Wright, London

Howard J 1992 Bach flower remedies for women. CW Daniel, Saffron Walden, Essex

House of Commons Health Committee 1992 Maternity services second report. HMSO, London

Hunt S, Symonds A 1995 The social meaning of midwifery. Macmillan, Basingstoke

Jeffery P, Jeffery R, Lyon A 1989 Labour pains and labour power. Zed Books, London

Jenkins MW, Pritchard MH 1993 Hypnosis: practical applications and theoretical considerations in normal labour. British Journal of Obstetrics and Gynaecology 100: 221–226

Jepson C 1989 Water: can it help in childbirth? Nursing Times 85(47): 74–75

Jordan B 1993 Birth in four cultures. Waveland Press, Illinois

Jowitt M 1993 Childbirth unmasked. Peter Wooller, Walford

Jurgens A, Meehan TC, Wilson HL 1987 Therapeutic touch as a nursing intervention. Holistic Nurse Practitioner 2(1): 1–13

Keller E, Bzdek VM 1986 Effects of therapeutic touch on tension and headache. Nursing Research 35(2): 101

Kitzinger S 1988 The midwife challenge. Pandora, London

Kramer NA 1990 Comparison of therapeutic touch and casual touch in stress reduction in hospitalised children. Paediatric Nursing 16: 483

Krieger D 1972 The response of in vivo human haemoglobin to an active healing therapy by direct laying-on of hands. Human Dimensions 1: 12–15

Krieger D 1974 Healing by the laying-on of hands as a facilitator of bioenergetic change. Psychoenergetic Systems 3(3): 121–129

Lawless J 1992 The encyclopedia of essential oils. Element, Dorset

Leap N 1992 The power of words. Nursing Times 88: 21 60–61

LeCron DA 1971 A complete guide to hypnosis. Harper & Row, New York

Leduc E 1989 The healing touch. American Journal of Nursing 14: 41–43

Levine B 1984 Use of hydrotherapy in reducing anxiety. Psychological Reports 515–526

McCandlish R, Renfrew M 1993 Immersion in water during labour and birth: the need for evaluation. Birth 20(20): 79–85

Mackey RB 1995 Discover the healing power of therapeutic touch. American Journal of Nursing 95(4): 26–32

MacRae J 1979 Therapeutic touch in practice. American Journal of Nursing 79(4): 664–665

MacRae J 1987 Therapeutic touch: a practical guide. Alfred A Knopf, Westminster, Maryland

Meehan MTC 1985 The effect of therapeutic touch on the experience of acute pain in postoperative patients. PhD thesis. New York University Dissertation Abstracts International 46(3): 795

Miller LA 1979 An explanation of therapeutic touch using the science of unitary man. Nursing Forum XVIII(3): 278–287

Milner I 1983 Water baths for pain relief in labour. Nursing Times 84(1): 39–40

Montagu A 1978 Touching: the human significance of the skin. Harper & Row, London

Morse JM, Park C 1988 Home birth and hospital deliveries: a comparison of the perceived painfulness of parturition. Research in Nursing and Health 11: 175–181

Newshaw G 1989 Therapeutic touch for symptom control in persons with AIDS. Holistic Nurse Practitioner 3(4): 45–51

Newton N, Fosheu D, Newton M 1966 Experimental inhibition of labour through environmental disturbance. Obstetrics and Gynaecology 27: 371–377

Nightingale C 1994 Waterbirth in practice. Modern Midwife 4(1): 15–19

Niven C 1994 Coping with labour pain: the midwife's role. In: Robinson S, Thompson A (eds) Midwife research and childbirth 3. Chapman & Hall, London, ch 5

Odent M 1983 Birth under water. Lancet 24(31): 1476–1477

Odent M 1984 Birth reborn – what birth can and should be. Souvenir, London

Olson M, Sneed N, Bonadonna R, Ratcliffe J, Dias J 1992 Therapeutic touch and post-hurricane Hugo stress. Journal of Holistic Nursing 10(2): 120

Parsons C 1994 Back care in pregnancy. Modern Midwife October 16–19

Payne MB 1989 The use of therapeutic touch with rehabilitation clients. Rehabilitation Nursing 14: 69–72

Quinn JF 1982 An investigation of the effects of therapeutic touch done without physical contact on state anxiety of hospitalised cardiovascular patients. PhD, New York University

Quinn JF 1989 Therapeutic touch as energy exchange: replication and extension. Nurse Science Quarterly 2(2): 79

Reed L, Norfolk L 1993 Aromatherapy in midwifery. International Journal of Alternative and Complementary Medicine 11(12): 15–17

Rich A 1977 Of woman born: motherhood as experience and institution. Virago, London

Rogers M 1980 In: Barrett EAM (ed) Visions of Rogers' science-based nursing. National League for Nursing Publications, New York

Rosa L 1998 A close look at therapeutic touch. Journal of the American Medical Association 279: 1005–1010

Royal College of Midwives 1989 Guidelines for midwives facing moral or ethical dilemmas. RCM, London

Rubin R 1963 Maternal touch. Nursing Outlook 11: 828–831

Sakala C 1988 Content of care by independent midwives: assistance with pain in labour and birth. Social Science and Medicine 26: 1141–1158

Sayre-Adams J 1994 Therapeutic touch: a nursing function. Nursing Standard 8(17): 25–28

Scarry E 1985 The body in pain: the making and unmaking of the world. Oxford University Press, Oxford

Sidenbladh E 1983 Waterbabies: Igor Tjarkovsky and his methods of delivering and training children in water. A & C Black, London

Simington JA 1993 Therapeutic touch for the elderly. Nurse Practitioner 18(11): 23–24

Simkin P 1995 Reducing pain and enhancing progress in labour: a guide to nonpharmacologic methods for maternity caregivers. Birth 22(3): 161–171

Simkin P, Dickerson K 1990 Control of pain in labour. In Enkin M et al (eds) Effective care in pregnancy. Oxford University Press, Oxford, pp 212–224

Stapleton H 1995 Herbal medicines for disorders of pregnancy. Modern Midwife Apr: 18–22

Sutcliffe J 1991 The complete book of relaxation techniques. Headline, London

Thayer MB 1990 Touching with intent: using therapeutic touch. Paediatric Nursing 16(1): 70–72

Tiran D, Mack S 1995 Complementary therapies for pregnancy and childbirth, 1st edn. Baillière Tindall, London, ch 10, p 222

Turton P 1989 Touch me, feel me, heal me. Nursing Times 85(19): 42–44

UKCC 1998 Midwives rules and code of practice. UKCC, London

Vadurro JF, Butts PA 1982 Reducing the anxiety and pain of childbirth through hypnosis. American Journal of Nursing 82: 620–623

Vincent Priya J 1992 Birth traditions and modern pregnancy care. Element, Shaftesbury

Wagner M 1986 Birth and power. In: Phaff J. (ed) Perinatal health services in Europe. Croom Helm, London, ch 16

Wine PM 1988 Superficial hypnosis – an aid to midwifery. Midwife, Health Visitor and Community Nurse 25: 518–524

Wirth D 1990 Non-contact therapeutic touch works, prove it! RN – Medical Economics at Montvale, NJ 59(12): 76

Wirth D 1993 Full thickness dermal wounds treated with non-contact therapeutic touch: a replication and extension. Complementary Therapies Medicine 1: 127–132

Wright TC 1995 Complementary therapies: touch of all kinds is therapeutic. Medical Economics 58(2): 61–64

8

Pharmacological methods of pain relief

Margaret Yerby

INTRODUCTION

Since the Peel Report (Department of Health 1970) women have increasingly had the opportunity of a wider choice of pharmacological preparations in

111

labour to assist with pain relief. At that time the report suggested that a woman should be offered a hospital bed for every birth; this altered the place of birth for the mother, from home to hospital. The midwife needed to develop new skills in the hospital as some tasks became more involved with electrical fetal heart monitoring and the development of more complex pain relief. The methods for administering pain preparations became more complex, needing the assistance of a medical practitioner. The whole process termed 'the medicalization of childbirth' brought many changes, some for the better, others not. Women were able to have a greater choice in the type of pain relief with more improved control of pain but sometimes at the expense of the progress of labour or the type of birth they had. The hospital environment undoubtedly altered the atmosphere of the birthing room as it was clinical and controlled and the woman consequently became more anxious (Haddard & Morris 1982). The National Birthday Trust Survey (NBT) 1990 (Chamberlain et al 1993) reported that anxiety was cited by 20% of women as the one thing that stopped them relaxing, restriction to bed and hospital surroundings were less important parameters.

Chapters 1 and 5 have outlined the historical events leading to the changes in the available pain relief for women. This chapter will address the physiological aspects of pain relief and the resultant effects on both mother and fetus or baby. The efficiency of each pharmacological medication will be evaluated against research findings, and women's views taken into account.

The Standards for the Administration of Medicines (UKCC (United Kingdom Central Council for Nursing, Midwifery and Health Visiting) 1992) and The Midwives Rules and Code of Practice (UKCC 1998) clearly give guidance in the use and handling of drugs given to the mother. At all times a midwife should be conversant with the unit or health authority policy regarding drugs but also be aware of her own competency in the administration of drugs and be able to acquire new skills in the use of such drugs if the need should arise (UKCC 1998). As new preparations are introduced she should acquire the information on the effects of medication and the possible side-effects, thus improving client care.

PHARMACOLOGICAL TERMS

Pharmacokinetics is the study of drug absorption, metabolism, distribution and excretion in the body. The processes are altered during pregnancy because of the physiological adaptation of maternal systems. The cardiac output increases in response to circulatory changes. Weight gain in pregnancy is caused in part by the growing fetus but also the changes in fluid within the body compartments which alters the distribution of drugs and plasma concentrations (de Swiet & Chamberlain 1992). The liver may not conjugate drugs so effectively in late pregnancy because of the increasing levels of progesterone and pregnanendiol which affect this pathway (Crawford & Rudofsky 1966, Burt 1971). The kidneys' increased blood supply may enhance their ability to excrete substances which are 'flow dependent'. This could assist in a more rapid excretion of drugs from both the mother and the fetus which could have a beneficial effect once metabolized (Reynolds 1991). Experimental data in relation to the excretion of anaesthetics and analgesia are contradictory. Pharmacodynamics is a term used when analysing how drugs affect the body systems, for example how analgesia in its various forms affects the nervous system. Knowledge of these changes is important when considering drug doses in pregnancy and the efficiency of the medication and its effect, and when considering that the fetus will also absorb and react to drugs administered. This is important in labour when giving analgesia because of the effects of the drug on the fetus as well as the physiological effects on maternal body systems and labour itself. It will also be important to consider the effects of the labour process on the woman's physiology and how she copes with the changing parameters of the labour and delivery of her baby.

WOMEN AND CHOICE

Childbirth preparation classes introduce women to the types of pain relief that are on offer in the unit in which they are going to have their baby. They may well make up their minds before the birth, but it is not until they experience pain that they may realize that the natural methods of coping with pain, such as relaxation or massage, may not be working for them. They then need to have a more effective pain-controlling medication. Many feel let down by their own body systems, particularly if they have wanted a natural birth without medications.

Comments from women who participated in the National Birthday Trust (NBT) Survey (Chamberlain et al 1993) bore witness to this by stating:

My labour was so different from my expectations that my preconceived intentions regarding pain relief became irrelevant (p 85)

and another felt let down:

I was disappointed with my ability to cope with the pain; perhaps I had unrealistic expectations (p 85)

It is impossible to estimate how labour pain will affect you until labour commences, there are so many dimensions to the pain experience. In the '1000 Mothers Survey', Morgan et al (1982) looked at mothers' satisfaction with pain relief and found that women who recalled their labours as 'nightmares' were women who had long labours and instrumental deliveries.

Although mothers in this survey with shorter normal labours had high pain scores they related better feelings of satisfaction immediately and one year later. It would appear that more severe pain is forgotten and milder more nagging pain and the experiences of longer labours with perhaps more interventions are less easily forgotten.

NITROUS OXIDE

Over the years the administration of inhalation analgesia for women in labour has been the simplest and possibly safest method of pain relief, easily portable for use in the home and self administered by the woman with the midwife supporting her. The gas has been mixed with oxygen to increase its safety and may be supplied in cylinders for ease of portability or as in most modern obstetric units piped to the delivery suites. At normal room temperatures the gases remain well mixed, but at temperatures of –8°C or below the gases separate leaving nitrous oxide at the bottom of the cylinder. Most community midwives would deliver fresh cylinders to the home as labour commenced thus eliminating the risk of having stored Entonox in too cold an environment and the potential of administering pure nitrous oxide instead of a 50% mixture with oxygen (Russell & Reynolds 1997). Before using a new cylinder to avoid such disasters inverting the cylinder would eliminate this problem.

Nitrous oxide, on its own known as 'laughing gas', which is a self explanatory side-effect, can be used effectively in labour if mixed with oxygen in a 50%–50% mixture (Entonox). It has a sedative, amnesic effect but not an analgesic effect in use. It may well cause hallucinations in some women if used over a long period of time. As it is self administered by the woman it will not cause unconsciousness, unless the woman becomes hypoxic. Although the analgesic effect is limited it is liked by many women because they remain in control. Its effects are quite rapid, commencing 20 seconds after administration with a maximum effect at 60 seconds, and it is essential that the breathing technique is correct, short panting breaths are not effective whereas deep breathing at the normal rate is effective (Moir 1986). To obtain effective relief from pain it should be inhaled before the contraction begins, then at the height of contraction when it is most painful it has had time to produce its effect.

Pharmacokinetics

Nitrous oxide may be termed a low-solubility anaesthetic agent, which in effect means that when inspired into the lungs the transfer from the alveoli into the blood stream reaches fast equilibrium with the inspired gas and acts rapidly, this conversely means that arterial pressure will fall rapidly and the gas will be expired rapidly (Rang et al 1995). In pregnancy if administered for anaesthetic purposes lower levels are required for effective unconscious levels than in the non-pregnant client, in part this is due to the increase in steroid hormones (Fujinaga & Badon 1995, Jayaram 1997). Entonox with a composition of 50% nitrous oxide and 50% oxygen, and self administered by the mother, will gain its effect rapidly. As consciousness declines the mouth piece or mask drops away from the woman's face and she will rapidly expire the gas from her system and regain consciousness again clearing the gas.

Nitrous oxide effects

The kinetic effect in the body depends on respiratory activity and alveolar absorption rate. A fit healthy person such as a woman in labour will get beneficial absorption and excretion with few side-effects, however there is complete absorption through the placenta (Carson 1996). The amount absorbed by the mother rapidly gains an equilibrium in the fetus but equally so it is also rapidly cleared from the fetal system when inhalation is stopped by the mother. Entonox has no effect on uterine contractility (Jayaram 1997). Modified respiratory effort in the mother may decrease uteroplacental perfusion to the fetus by constriction of the placental vessels; this may occur when she commences self administration because of an inadequate technique, and breathing patterns alter (Gamsu 1993).

In the NBT survey (Chamberlain et al 1993) Entonox was available in 99% of the units included in the study. In the questionnaire 60% of women had used Entonox and it was the most frequently used form of analgesia, except where the epidural rate was higher than 50%. The majority of the women who used it rated it as 'useful' or 'highly useful'.

Occupational hazards of nitrous oxide

It has long been identified that there may be an increased risk of abortion and low birth weight and preterm birth in low dose exposure to nitrous oxide in personnel who work in operating theatres and dental surgeries (Holson et al 1995, Rowland et al 1995, Axelsson et al 1996). Midwives could be put at risk during pregnancy while working, as it has been suggested that exposure during nitrous oxide use in non-vented rooms could pose a greater risk to reproductive health because gases are unable to escape (Rowland et al 1995). However small the risk it should be taken into consideration with the work environment as a whole, as midwives work long shifts with few breaks. Axelsson et al (1996) studied shift patterns of midwives in Sweden and found that odds ratios for the risk of spontaneous abortion vs contact with nitrous oxide was not associated with a higher risk, but that long shift patterns and shortage of staff increased the risk of abortion before 13 weeks of pregnancy. One study monitored the exposure of midwives to nitrous oxide gas and showed that exposure levels exceeded the recommended levels in the USA, Sweden and the UK (Mills et al 1996). In the light of this research perhaps we should consider the length of shift patterns of our pregnant colleagues and limit their exposure to nitrous oxide in the labour ward.

OPIOIDS AND THEIR DERIVATIVES

Opioid analgesics include the morphine-like substances derived from the opium poppy (*Papaver somniferum*) that induce 'euphoria, analgesia and sleep' (Rang et al 1995). They have been widely used in midwifery for women in labour since the 1950s (Bradford & Chamberlain 1995), this is mainly because they are readily available and easy to administer by intramuscular injection. They may be given by a midwife under Standing Orders in the delivery suite without the requirement for a prescription from a medical practitioner (Reynolds 1993a). The derivative most commonly used in the 1990s is pethidine (meperidine in America), which is a synthetic substance shorter acting than morphine with the effect of producing euphoria and sometimes dysphoria. Its pain-relieving properties in labour are disputed by many women who do not like the side-effect it produces. In the NBT Survey 1990 (Chamberlain et al 1993) as the labour length increased so the use of pethidine decreased and women turned to more effective methods of pain relief such as epidural. Olofsson et al (1996) compared the pain-relieving properties of morphine and pethidine in a double-blind randomized trial. Their sample was of 20 multiparous women, ten in each group. The women had high pain scores and were well sedated but woke to uterine contractions. Their conclusions were that they felt it unethical to use pethidine or morphine as a pain-relieving agent as it was only useful for its sedative affect.

Pethidine binds to receptor proteins to diffuse through cell membranes to exert its effect within the central nervous system. Its action at the cellular level alters potassium and calcium channel exchange in the neuronal membrane, thus calming the excitability of the nerve as it reacts to the pain-producing substances. It acts on efferent nerve pathways descending from the brain at the dorsal horn, thus playing a role in the gate theory of pain at the spinal column level (Rang et al 1995, Scrutton 1997). It is metabolized by the liver to norpethidine (normeperidine in America) by a process termed n-demethylation, which produces a substance that is half the potency of the original substance and has a stimulant convulsive effect (Jayaram 1997). In the neonate both pethidine and its metabolite have a respiratory depressant effect. Metabolism is very dependent on the efficiency of the liver's blood flow (Reynolds 1991) and thus would be dependent on good liver function and circulatory efficiency. It has been found that in the pregnant state there may be more unmetabolized substances excreted by the kidneys, which possibly shows the efficiency of the maternal systems and its adaptation to pregnancy to effect adequate excretion of drugs.

Fetal effects

Diffusion across the placenta occurs readily and will easily obtain an equilibrium with maternal levels. This does depend on the lipid solubility of the drug and its molecular weight. The lower pH levels of the fetus to the mother would suggest a greater transfer of the active drug (Low 1963, Burt 1971). The route of the administration is also important when considering fetal effect. Following an intravenous dose of pethidine it has been found in the cord blood within 2 minutes (Briggs et al 1994). Tests on maternal and fetal blood following the administration of intramuscular pethidine showed that 2 hours after administration pethidine began to pass back to the mother via the placenta (Cawthra 1986). Undoubtedly pethidine passes from mother to fetus very readily as does the metabolite norpethidine and this is dose dependent. The fetus will also produce norpethidine and the levels in the fetal circulation may be higher in the fetus than in the mother. The fetus may be more susceptible to the effects of this type of medication because of the immaturity of the blood–brain barrier and the fetal bypass of the liver where it would normally be metabolized (Burt 1971). When the birth of the baby follows within 2–5 hours of administration there may well be more respiratory depression in the neonate; although this is the peak time for neonatal effect it may also occur if delivery occurs prior to 2 hours (Belfrage et al 1981). The plasma half-life of pethidine in the maternal systems is 3–4 hours whereas the levels in the infants' plasma are 13–23 hours with the metabolite norpethidine still being present at 62 hours (Righard & Alade 1990). This has been shown to have implications on the infant's neurobehavioral state at birth and up to 3 days post birth.

Antagonists

Naloxone is commonly given where there is an observed effect such as low Apgar scores or difficulty in establishing breathing following the administration of pethidine in the neonate. It is an antagonist blocking the receptors that pethidine binds to, thus blocking the effect of pethidine and its consequent depressant effect on respiration. It is safe for the neonate and may be given via the intramuscular route in doses of 1 mg per kg of body weight. The baby has not usually been weighed at this point and therefore an estimation of drug–weight ratio has to be made. Any treatment to improve neonatal condition following birth may well require medical intervention. This would require the baby's removal from its mother and interference with the immediate postnatal mother interaction altering the neonatal response to its mother and creating anxiety for the parents. Scrutton (1997) suggests that if the fetus has been exposed to high levels of pethidine or its derivatives during pregnancy as in a drug-abusing mother, naloxone may induce fitting and severe withdrawal symptoms and should not be used in this situation.

Pethidine usage and subsequent infant feeding

A study of babies who were placed skin to skin with their mothers and a control group who were not, instigated their breastfeeding patterns within 1 hour. Just over half of the mothers were given pethidine (*n*=40/72); of these infants it was noted that 25 did not suck at all and it was felt that pethidine should be used with caution in the light of these findings (Righard & Alade 1990). These researchers felt that delivery room routines were important in the instigation of the first feed and this first contact often sets the scene for successful breastfeeding patterns in the future. Pethidine is excreted in breast milk and when compared to morphine is more readily excreted there than morphine because it is more lipid soluble (Wittels 1990, Jayram 1997).

THE USE OF LOCAL ANAESTHETICS

Midwives administer local anaesthetics during the course of delivery to prevent the pain of perineal trauma prior to an episiotomy. Most units will have a written policy (Standing Orders) which enables this to be undertaken without a prescription in specific doses as specified by the unit consultants and pharmacists. Lignocaine is the commonly used agent which is given in strengths of 1% or 0.5%, the dose being 5 ml and 10 ml respectively (Sweet 1997). During administration it is important to protect the fetal presenting part, as accidental injection of the fetus could lead to 'apnoea, loss of muscle tone and fixed dilated pupils' following birth (Kim et al 1979, Briggs et al 1994). The effect upon the fetus depends on the dose of drug and the time the fetus is exposed to the drug's properties. It has been shown that the neonate is still excreting the drug and its metabolite at 48 hours post delivery when lignocaine has been injected into the perineum at the crowning of the fetal head (Philipson 1984, Reynolds 1993b).

Kinetic effects

Lignocaine is relatively short acting in comparison to bupivacaine, and is more rapidly absorbed from the tissues because it has a vasodilatory effect (Russell & Reynolds 1997). Local anaesthetics block sensation in the tissues by being absorbed into the nerve and preventing sodium flux in the nerve, and thus halting the action potential and membrane activity (Rang et al 1995) (Fig. A.5). They are absorbed into the tissues and the circulatory system which enables metabolism and excretion from the maternal system (British Medical Association and the Royal Pharmacological Society 1998). In the healthy mother during pregnancy lignocaine is distributed well within the tissues. It is essential that the tissues have a good blood circulation to aid the drug's excretion, but it is also important not to inject a local anaesthetic into a vein or major blood vessel. This may cause convulsions and respiratory and cardiovascular collapse and in some an allergic reaction which is rare (Rang et al 1995). The unwanted side-effects are produced by the local anaesthetic escaping into the general circulation.

Bupivacaine used for epidural administration may have an opioid added to decrease the dose of bupivacaine. This will prevent a motor block which would otherwise render the woman incapable of movement in her lower limbs. The consequence of the heavier block increases bladder function problems and instrumental deliveries (Rang et al 1995, O'Sullivan 1997).

In a study to compare the use of fentanyl with bupivacaine or bupivacaine alone, James et al (1998) found that there was greater client satisfaction with less incidence of assisted births in a group who were administered fentanyl with bupivacaine. The second stages of these women was also shorter, with a $P=0.0003$ and a 95% confidence interval.

EPIDURAL ANAESTHESIA

The advent of total pain relief in labour has rescued many desperate women from a painful protracted labour, the midwife only needs to observe the effect that a fully effective epidural has on the demeanour of her client to understand this. In Chapter 3 it was discussed that pain alters the physiological response increasing heart rate and adrenaline levels, and psychologically fear can be detrimental to the whole process of labour. An epidural is the only complete type of pain relief available that effectively blocks labour pain, but it is an invasive technique requiring an expert anaesthetist for its administration. The midwife needs to monitor both the mother and the fetus more closely and particularly during top-ups. It requires some degree of understanding as to its advantages and disadvantages from the client's viewpoint. It enables women to maintain control and dignity which is all important in the labour process (Mander

1997). Midwives found it difficult to come to terms with this form of pain relief in its early days of use because it required the expertise of the anaesthetist for siting and for further top-ups as labour progressed, thus seemingly taking control out of their hands and altering the course of labour. In the 1970s high induction rates led to higher caesarean section rates and many of these labours were also epidural labours. Because of this many researchers set out to prove that it was not the effect of the epidural. It is suggested by Chamberlain et al (1993) that 83% of women have total pain relief and only 3% report no pain relief. The fact that the epidural rate in 1998 was rising in most maternity units is not surprising, as many women relate their amount of satisfaction after experiencing a totally pain-free labour. However its acceptance has enabled the decline of general anaesthetic use for most caesarean sections which has improved many women's and partners' experience of a difficult labour and failed normal birth, and the prevention of the associated deaths from anaesthesia (Morgan 1987).

Epidural induction

No woman should have an epidural, which is an invasive technique, accessing major areas within the lumbar spine and the injection of a potentially dangerous medication, without understanding the risks involved. They must make an informed choice. How good is that choice when they are in pain and desperate for relief from it? Do they understand the true problems of an epidural when in so much pain when it is explained to them under these circumstances (Russell 1997)? It is important for the midwife to record such discussions with the woman in the notes and Russell (1997) suggests that the anaesthetists could also sign in the notes that this has been done (UKCC 1992). Many of these aspects should be part of parent education classes when the woman is not in labour and is able to 'digest' the information with a clarity of mind not dulled by the environment or the fear and anticipation that ultimately overcomes women when labour commences (Crawford 1985, Robertson 1994, Russell 1997). A midwife will be at the forefront of care and will be able to allay their fears. Women may be reticent to choose an epidural when they have previously opted for other pain relief which has then been ineffective. They may feel as though they have failed because they changed their mind. However on some occasions it is the midwife who is reluctant to suggest an epidural because she is aware of the side-effects it may produce disrupting the course of normal labour. The anaesthetist will often not commence an epidural at full dilatation (Flint 1997). Whichever scenario is presented it is the woman's choice.

Anatomy of epidural analgesia

As has been discussed earlier, pain alters the normal physiological mechanisms of the body. The injection of bupivacaine into the two or three lumbar spaces between the vertebrae will block sensation to the areas of thoracic 10, 11 and 12 and below to the lower sacral segments. This has to block autonomic pathways in order for pain relief to occur. Motor pathways may also be blocked but these nerve pathways are more resistant to the actions of bupivacaine. This acts by inhibiting action potential within the A delta and B fibres which transfer pain from the uterus to the dorsal horn of the spinal column. The spinal cord is protected by the meninges and the surrounding vertebral spinal processes of the spinal column. At the level of lumbar 1 the spinal cord becomes the cauda equina which is a collection of nerve roots, lumbar, sacral and coccygeal. This, as the Latin suggests, resembles a horse's tail (Thibodeau 1990) (Fig. A.6). To gain access to the epidural space increased flexion is required to open the space between the vertebrae. The ligamentum flavum is a tough ligament which has to be overcome prior to insertion of the needle into the epidural space which is a potential space, approximately 4 mm thick at the level of insertion, containing blood vessels, nerve roots and fat (Moir 1986, Russell & Reynolds 1997) (Fig. A.7). It extends from the base of the skull to the sacrococcygeal membrane and is continuous, although where epidural analgesia fails it is thought that there may be a fold in the membrane diverting the flow of analgesic away from the nerves (Russell & Reynolds 1997).

The position of the woman during the procedure is quite important and a matter of preference of the anaesthetist. However the left lateral position favours improved uterine perfusion to the placenta. The upright position for the woman is more natural and pleasant, but may be unpleasant later in labour because of sacral pressure and it is not as easy to remain really still for the insertion of the needle. Whichever position is used good flexion of the lumbar spine is essential (Russell 1997). The midwife in the delivery room should remain close to and support the woman both physically and psychologically throughout the procedure. She should also maintain observation of maternal and fetal conditions while the epidural is commenced and maintain her record keeping of these events. Partners are also fearful at this point and may well be able to assist by helping their partner with the use of Entonox which may still be required to give adequate pain relief in order to maintain position while the procedure is carried out.

MATERNAL HEALTH AND EPIDURAL COMPLICATIONS

It is often recommended that women with raised blood pressure would benefit from epidural pain relief in labour because of the potential for the procedure to lower blood pressure as the resultant effect on the sympathetic nervous system. It is important to test the level of blood platelets prior to the procedure, as a low platelet count could result in an increased risk of an epidural haematoma. Blood pressure is auscultated frequently during labour but should be taken immediately prior to the induction of the epidural to assess baseline and an intravenous infusion should be commenced. Although it is quite common to preload with intravenous fluid to prevent hypovolaemia, it has been suggested that this could effect uterine contractility if saline is used (Cheek et al 1996). Cheek et al (1996) examined the relationship of three groups of spontaneously labouring women. The groups had either no preload, 500 ml preload or 1000 ml preload of normal saline intravenously. The uterine contractions were measured with an intrauterine pressure catheter. There appeared to be no hypotensive attacks in the non-preload group but a decrease in uterine contractility in the preload groups. Although the aetiology of this action was difficult to explain, physiologically two answers were proposed. First, that the local anaesthetic contained a proportion of adrenaline which has been known to affect the myometrial activity (Lederman et al 1978). Second, that the increase of fluid pressure on the heart increased atrial natriuretic peptide (ANP) and this substance in rats has been shown to decrease uterine activity (Cheek et al 1996). The preload fluid of choice in most maternity units is Hartman's solution; however the preload solution would still affect the pressure sensitivity in the heart producing higher levels of ANP with the same result on the uterine activity. Spinal deformity or spinal injury may affect the available access for induction or may affect the position of membranes and nerves if prior surgery has taken place but is not a contraindication to an epidural. Other aspects which may contraindicate the use of the technique for pain relief would be general sepsis, local sepsis, hypovolaemia, allergy to the drugs used or coagulopathy, either pathological or drug induced (Telfer 1997).

Physiological effects of the epidural on the body systems

The effect on the body mechanisms in labour are all encompassing and can be divided between the pain-relieving properties and the general effect of the epidural on the body systems. The immediate effect for the women should be total relief from pain and an ability to relax and smile again, to hold a conversation with her partner and the midwife and to enjoy her labour and anticipate the birth without fear. The physiological effects on her body are such that noradrenaline and adrenaline levels are decreased resulting in a decreased pulse rate and lowered blood pressure (May 1994). Decreasing the levels of these substances may aid uterine contractility; Lederman et al (1978) suggested that high adrenaline levels lengthened labour by diminishing uterine activity. Hyperventilation is decreased because the woman is relaxed, which immediately helps maternal and consequently fetal blood gases to return to normal pregnancy levels. Cortisol levels are decreased which may decrease the secretion of adrenaline, which in turn will calm the woman and permit the labour to continue (Jowitt 1993). Stress itself however can be a driving force increasing beta-endorphins, our natural opioids, and assisting in a natural pain-relieving process.

Sympathetic nervous system

The effect on the autonomic nervous system produces a vasodilatory effect in the peripheral circulation by blocking the sympathetic nerves. This is shown by warmth and non-sweating in the lower extremities, a good sign that the epidural is working. However pooling of the circulation in the periphery may cause hypotension, as there is a loss of peripheral resistance in the lower limbs. Aortocaval compression is always a risk from 20 weeks of gestation, therefore position in labour is important and the left lateral tilt would be favoured at all times, including vaginal examinations. Custom and practice show all personnel performing vaginal examinations in the supine position – perhaps we should change our practice? Blocking the sympathetic system should in theory improve fetal blood flow (Reynolds 1993b).

Unwanted side-effects

Bladder

The avoidance of damage to the bladder during labour must be prevented at all costs and the woman in labour must be encouraged to void urine every 2–3 hours. This only becomes difficult when the sensation of a full bladder is absent, and then many women find that it is difficult to micturate. A full bladder may lead to postnatal atonia and consequent transient incontinence, add to this a higher incidence of instrumental delivery and trauma and this increases the problem (Hawkins et al 1995, Russell 1997).

Progress of labour

In considering why the length of the first stage of labour should be influenced by the epidural it should first be hypothesized as to why women have asked for an epidural in the first place. Were they feeling more pain because of an abnormal fetal position and was the labour longer to begin with, was uterine activity inefficient before the epidural was commenced? Thorp & Breedlove (1996) found the research conflicting as the research designs made it difficult to compare studies, but some studies did show that the length of labour was longer compared to control groups.

Lack of oxytocin at second stage of labour

Goodfellow et al (1983) studied blood samples of primigravidae in the second stage of labour and at crowning, the two groups either had epidurals or Pethidine with Stemetil (prochlorperazine) and nitrous oxide. Blood samples had similar oxytocin levels on both occasions until data was paired and there seemed a significant rise of oxytocin in the non-epidural group. This research compared previous research data which had similar findings. It would seem that the analgesic block diminishes the Ferguson reflex (Ferguson 1941, Goodfellow et al 1983), which provides the uterus with an expelling force as the fetal head stretches the cervix to full dilatation and gives the mother the urge to push. Crawford (1982) suggests that the paralysis of the pelvic floor muscles also prevents rotation of the fetal presenting part to the anterior causing delay in the second stage of labour. The abdominal muscles are also affected in this way and the woman has no desire to push because she is pain and sensation free. It would seem to be good policy to instigate the use of an oxytocin infusion to augment the second stage to prevent the incidence of forceps delivery in the woman with an epidural, and to delay pushing until the fetal head is visible (Thorp & Breedlove 1996).

Rise in maternal temperature

A rise in the maternal temperature may be caused by the disruption of sweating, thus the diminishing of a natural physiological response to overheating (Thorp & Nielson 1996). It would seem that core temperature is adversely affected by epidural analgesia but the mechanism is unclear (Camann et al 1991). The effect on subsequent care could be quite significant if the rise in temperature is undefined and there is a resultant need to investigate both the mother and infant for a site of infection. This creates intervention in an otherwise normal delivery of a healthy infant, altering the course of postnatal recovery and care and creating unnecessary anxiety for the parents.

Complications

In choosing an epidural for the relief of pain in labour women are immediately increasing the need for technological intervention; the procedure itself is not without hazards but in experienced hands this should not be a problem. The need for intensive observation by labour ward midwives is important and for them to be able to perform epidural top-ups and indeed to have an on-call anaesthetist is essential medical back up. True life-threatening occurrences rarely are seen, hypotension being avoided with good positioning and increase of intravenous fluids. The accidental induction of a higher nerve block than thoracic 10 in labour is unusual but higher blocks could create breathing problems and a subsequent need for resuscitation. The observation of maternal condition is important at all times; in particular a tingling tongue, which could be a symptom following the injection of local anaesthetic into a vein and may need immediate resuscitation and possible ventilation. This could also potentially occur if accidental puncture of the dura occurred and the dose inadvertently injected into the subarachnoid space. The required amount of bupivacaine for dural analgesia is much higher than required for spinal anaesthesia and would result in a profound spinal block (Russell 1997).

Dural tap and long-term risk

Occasionally a dural tap occurs at the induction of the epidural with the consequence of loss of pressure in the cerebrospinal fluid. In some women this may cause a headache in labour or postnatally. Although disconcerting this can be treated with an autologous blood patch, 20 ml of the client's blood is used by injecting near the site of epidural to seal the hole in the dura (Crawford 1980, Reynolds 1997). It is important to rest the woman prior to the procedure and following the procedure, as this will minimize headache and the amount of cerebrospinal fluid leakage at the puncture site.

In attempting to calculate the long-term risk of epidural a questionnaire was sent to 203 units in the UK. Responses from 86 units were analysed and revealed 108 reports of complications out of a total of 505 000 epidural blocks (Scott & Hibbard 1990), of these only five caused permanent damage. A study by Holdcroft et al (1995) in the North West Thames area found that there appeared to be one in 2530 serious neurological complications associated with pregnancy. One in 13 007 had a prolonged paraesthaesia along a nerve root. Seven in 19 women had a continuing neurological disability for 1 year. Unfortunately it is the serious damage caused by any medical intervention that 'hits the headlines' and causes women concern, particularly in the popular press as accounts may be coloured by emotion and public opinion masking medical facts and causes.

Long-term backache

Backache is a very common problem in pregnancy and this may increase with the alteration of posture and the weight of the baby on ligaments and joints. MacArthur et al (1990) used data over a 7-year period from one maternity unit to investigate the association with an epidural and backache following birth. Backache was reported by 1634 (69%) women for over a year. Statistical analysis showed a relationship between backache and epidural for pain relief for normal labour but not for caesarean section. The researchers' explanation for this suggests that the postural stress during labour and the lack of sensation could put unusual strain on bones and ligaments because mobility and sensation are lacking. Other researchers have tried to quantify the type of backache and its association with other factors (Russell et al 1993). An analysis of 753 primiparae was made over a period of a year, these women had not complained of back pain before delivery. A questionnaire was completed by the women and they were then asked to attend an assessment clinic to quantify the back pain which they complained of following the birth of their baby. Their findings were similar to MacArthur et al (1990) and in the final follow-up of 36 women who attended an outpatient clinic to assess their back pain there seemed to be no difference in those who did or did not have an epidural. As can be seen by the figures, many women declined a follow-up clinic. Most back pain could be attributed to poor posture and the women had just blamed the form of pain relief they had in childbirth. It was also interesting to consider that these women had not considered their pain bad enough prior to the investigation to seek medical advice. Breen and associates (1994) found no association with epidural use and long-term backache and suggested that back pain initiated during pregnancy would be expected to continue postnatally and if an epidural was used this was the reason why the women felt they had pain. As the research data broadens in the long-term backache argument, there does not seem to be a link with either epidural or profound motor block from an epidural on back pain (Russell et al 1996).

COMBINED SPINAL (CSE) AND EPIDURAL; ALSO TERMED MOBILE EPIDURAL

One of the problems involved in the use of local anaesthetics is their effect on motor control and the ability of the woman to move around freely if she so wishes. Modern epidurals are beginning to use lower dose local analgesics such as a combination of bupivacaine and fentanyl with fewer side-effects and minimal motor block.

A group of anaesthetists at Queen Charlotte's Hospital (Collis et al 1993) developed the mobile epidural which involved a small dose of local anaesthetic into the subarachnoid space prior to inserting the normal epidural catheter and giving a further dose in the normal way. The needle was very much smaller than the large gauge Tuohy needle required for the normal epidural and is passed down the Tuohy needle and enters the subarachnoid space. When cerebrospinal fluid appears at the end of the needle, the dose of plain bupivacaine 2.5 mg and fentanyl 25 µg in 2 ml normal saline is given, the needle withdrawn and the epidural catheter inserted in the normal way. Intravenous Hartman's solution 1000 ml is used for a preload. Once blood pressure and fetal monitoring are satisfactory the woman is permitted to walk around with an attendant. The intravenous Hartman's solution is then discontinued. Prior to mobilization the anaesthetist tests the block by the warmth of the periphery for the sympathetic action, and motor control is gauged by a straight-leg raise against resistance. The first epidural top-up may be performed by an anaesthetist and subsequent doses by the midwife, on average these are required at 50-minute intervals. The average time of full pain relief occurred within 5 minutes in this study of 300 consecutive CSE at Queen Charlotte's (Collis et al 1993). Women reported liking this type of epidural because it gave them freedom to walk around. Many women did not walk far, around their rooms or short distances along the corridor. They reported that although they did not use alternative positions for delivery they felt they could have done so. They also commented on the fact that they were better able to push as they had more sensation as the fetal head descended on to the perineum.

CONCLUSION

It would seem the more invasive the analgesic, the more side-effects and problems that may be created by its use. However the most important factor is safety and that the woman chooses the pain relief that she needs and likes. No one wants to experience intense pain even for a process that is physiological. The CSE does seem to offer some of the answers except that there may be the added risk of infection when puncturing the dura. It is an effective method to relieve pain quickly and women can be mobile if they want to (Elton et al 1997). Research must continue to achieve optimum effective pain relief for women in labour in the most efficient safe manner. Women need to be informed of the options they may take and be realistically

Useful resources

◆ http://yakshlab.ucsd.edu/
◆ Broad spectrum of research into pain physiology and physiology of analgesia. Based in the University of California: Director TL Yakshi, San Diego
◆ http://www.rcoa.ac.uk/
◆ Royal College of Anaesthetists web page

informed of these options before they reach labour when, because of pain, their mind can be somewhat clouded by the events which overcome them and thus they are unable to make an informed choice.

ANNOTATED BIBLIOGRAPHY

Banister C 1997 The midwife's pharmacopeia. Books for Midwives Press, Hale, Cheshire

A very readable book useful for quick reference and well applied to the drugs used by the midwife.

Briggs G, Freeman R, Yaffe S (eds) 1998 Drugs in pregnancy and lactation. 5th edn. Lippincott, Williams and Wilkins

A very comprehensive textbook with drugs fully discussed and referenced in relation to fetal and neonatal risk.

British Medical Association and the Royal Pharmaceutical Society of Great Britain 1999 British National Formulary, no 37. Pharmaceutical Press, Oxon

A book found in all hospitals, a vast reference volume for all drugs in all aspects of care and for all conditions. There is a large appendix which includes drugs for pregnancy. Issued twice yearly so always up to date.

Coustan D, Mochizuki TK 1998 Handbook for prescribing medications during pregnancy, 3rd edn. Lippincott Williams and Wilkins, Baltimore

A book of interest to midwives but as the title suggests concentrates on the prescription of medications, a useful book for ward reference.

REFERENCES

Axelsson G, Ahlborg G Jr, Bodin L 1996 Shift work nitrous oxide, and spontaneous abortion among Swedish midwives. Occupational and Environmental Medicine 53: 374–378

Belfrage P, Boreus LO, Hartvig P, Irestedt L, Raabe N 1981 Neonatal depression after obstetrical analgesia with pethidine. The role of the injection-delivery time interval and plasma concentrations of pethidine and norpethidine. Acta Obstetrica et Gynecologica Scandinavica 60: 43–49

Bradford N, Chamberlain G 1995 Pain relief in childbirth. Harper Collins, London

Briggs GG, Freeman RK, Yaffe SJ 1994 Drugs in pregnancy and lactation, 4th edn. Williams and Wilkins, Baltimore

British Medical Association and Royal Pharmacological Society of Great Britain 1998 British National Formulary no 35. Pharmaceutical Press, Oxon, p 25

Breen TW, Ransil BJ, Groves PA, Oriol NE 1994 Factors associated with back pain after childbirth. Anaesthesiology 81: 29–34

Burt RAP 1971 The fetal and maternal pharmacology of some of the drugs used in the relief of pain in labour. British Journal of Anaesthesia 43: 824–833

Camann WR, Horvet LA, Hughes N, Badar AM, Datta S 1991 Maternal temperature regulation during extradural analgesia for labour. British Journal of Anaesthesia 67: 565–568

Carson R 1996 The administration of analgesics. Modern Midwife 6(11): 14–16

Cawthra AM 1986 The use of pethidine in labour. Midwives Chronicle and Nursing Notes Aug: 178–181

Chamberlain G, Wraight A, Steer P 1993 Pain and its relief in childbirth. Churchill Livingstone, Edinburgh

Cheek TG, Samuels P, Miller F, Tobin M, Gutsche BB 1996 Normal saline iv. fluid decreases uterine activity in active labour. British Journal of Anaesthesia 77: 632–635

Collis RE, Baxandall ML, Srikantharajah ID, Edge G, Kadim MY, Morgan BM 1993 Mobility during labour with combined analgesia. Lancet 341: 767–768

Crawford JS 1980 Experiences with epidural blood patch. Anaesthesia 35: 513–515

Crawford JS 1982 The effect of epidural block on the progress of labour. In: Studd J (ed) Progress in obstetrics and gynaecology, vol 2. Churchill Livingstone, Edinburgh, ch 9

Crawford JS 1985 The midwife's contribution to epidural analgesia for labour and delivery. Midwifery 1: 24–31

Crawford JS, Rudofsky S 1966 Some alterations in the pattern of drug metabolism associated with pregnancy, oral contraceptives and the newly born. British Journal of Anaesthesia 38: 446

Department of Health 1970 Domiciliary and maternity bed needs, Report of the Sub-committee of the Standing Midwifery and Maternity Advisory Committee (Peel Report). HMSO, London

de Swiet M, Chamberlain G 1992 Basic science in obstetrics and gynaecology, 2nd edn. Churchill Livingstone, Edinburgh

Elton CD, Ali P, Mushambi MC 1997 'Walking extradurals' in labour: a step forward? British Journal of Anaesthesia 79: 551–553

Ferguson JKW 1941 A study of the intact uterus at term. Surgery, Gynaecology and Obstetrics 73: 359–366

Flint C 1997 Do you want an epidural? Midirs, Midwifery Digest 4(1): 60–61

Fujinaga M, Baden JM 1995 Maternal and fetal effects of anaesthesia. In: Thomas EJ, Cohen PJ (eds) Wylie and Churchill Davidson's a practice of anaesthesia, 6th edn. Edward Arnold, London, ch 21

Gamsu H 1993 The effect of pain relief on the baby. In: Chamberlain G, Wraight A, Steer P (eds) Pain and its relief in childbirth. Churchill Livingstone, Edinburgh, ch 9

Goodfellow CF, Hull MGR, Swabb DF, Dogterom J, Buijs RM 1983 Oxytocin deficiency at delivery with epidural analgesia. British Journal of Obstetrics and Gynaecology 90: 214–219

Haddard PF, Morris NF 1982 The relationship between maternal anxiety to the events in labour. Journal of Obstetrics and Gynaecology 3: 94–97

Hawkins JL, Hess KR, Kubicek MA, Joyce TH, Morrow 1995 A re-evaluation of the association between instrumental delivery and epidural analgesia. Regional Analgesia 20: 50–56

Holdcroft A, Gibberd FB, Hargrove RL, Hawkins DF, Dellaportas CI 1995 Neurological complications associated with pregnancy. British Journal of Anaesthesia 75: 522–526

Holson RR, Bates HK, LaBorde JB, Hansen DK 1995 Behavioural teratology and dominant lethal evaluation of nitrous oxide exposure in rats. Neurotoxicology and Teratology 17: 583–592

James KS, McGrady E, Qusim I, Patrick A 1998 Comparison of epidural bolus administration of 0.25% bupivacaine and 0.1% bupivacaine with 0.0002% fentanyl for analgesia during labour. British Journal of Anaesthesia 81: 507–510

Jayaram A 1997 Practical obstetric pharmacology. In: Dewan D, Hood A (eds) Practical obstetrics anaesthesia. WB Saunders, London, p 76

Jowitt M 1993 Childbirth unmasked. Harnells, Bodmin, Cornwall

Kim WY, Pomerance JJ, Miller AA 1979 Lidocaine intoxication in a new-born following local anaesthesia for episiotomy. Paediatrics 64: 643–645

Lederman RP, Lederman E, Work B, MaCann D 1978 The relationship of maternal anxiety, plasma catecholamines, and plasma cortisol to the progression in labour. American Journal of Gynecology 1: 495–500

Low JA 1963 Acid base assessment of the fetus in the normal obstetric patient. Obstetrics and Gynaecology 22: 15

MacArthur C, Lewis M, Knox EG, Crawford JS 1990 Epidural and long term backache after childbirth. British Medical Journal 301(Jul): 9–12

Mander R 1997 Pain in childbearing and its control. Blackwell Scientific, Oxford

May A 1994 Epidurals for childbirth. Oxford University Press, London

Mills GH, Singh D, Longan M et al 1996 Nitrous oxide exposure in the labour ward. International Journal of Obstetric Anaesthesia 5: 160–164

Moir DD 1986 Pain relief in labour, 5th edn. Churchill Livingstone, Edinburgh

Morgan BM 1987 Mortality and anaesthesia. In: Morgan BM (ed) Foundations of Obstetric Anaesthesia. Farrand Press, London, pp 255–270

Morgan BM, Bulpitt CJ, Clifton CA, Lewis P 1982 Analgesia and satisfaction in childbirth. Lancet 9 Oct: 808–810

Olofsson CH, Ekblom A, Ekman-Ordeberg G, Helm AH, Irestedt L 1996 Lack of analgesic effect of systemically administered morphine or pethidine for labour pain. British Journal of Obstetrics and Gynaecology 103: 968–972

O'Sullivan G 1997 Epidural analgesia in labour: recent developments. British Journal of Midwifery 5: 555–556

Philipson EH, Kuhnert BR, Syracuse CD 1984 Maternal, fetal and neonatal lidocaine levels following local perineal infiltration. American Journal of Obstetrics and Gynecology 149: 403–407

Rang HP, Dale MM, Ritter JM 1995 Pharmacology, 3rd edn. Churchill Livingstone, Edinburgh

Reynolds F 1991 Pharmacokinetics. In: Clinical physiology in obstetrics. Blackwell Scientific, Oxford, ch 20, p 31

Reynolds F 1993a Pain relief in labour: a review. British Journal of Obstetrics and Gynaecology 100: 979–983

Reynolds F 1993b Effects on the baby of maternal analgesia and anaesthesia. WB Saunders, London

Reynolds F (1997) They think it's all over. In: Reynolds F (ed) Pain relief in labour. BMJ Publishing Group, London, ch 12

Righard L, Alade MO 1990 Effect of delivery rooms routines on the success of breast-fed infants. Lancet 336: 1105–1107

Robertson A 1994 Empowering women. Australian Print Group, Australia

Rowland AS, Baird DD, Shore DL, Weinberg CR, Savitz DA, Wilcox AJ 1995 Nitrous oxide and spontaneous abortion in female dental assistants. American Journal of Epidemiology 141: 531–538

Russell R 1997 Practical procedures. In: Reynolds F (ed) Pain relief in labour. BMJ Publishing Group, London, ch 10

Russell R, Groves P, Taub N, O'Dowd J, Reynolds F 1993 Assessing long term backache after childbirth. British Medical Journal 306: 1299–1303

Russell R, Reynolds F 1997 Neuroscientific aspects. In: Reynolds F (ed) Pain relief in labour. BMJ Publishing Group, London, ch 7

Russell R, Dundas R, Reynolds F 1996 Long term backache after childbirth: prospective search for causative factors. British Medical Journal 312: 1384–1388

Scott DB, Hibbard BM 1990 Serious non-fatal complications associated with extradural block in obstetric practice. British Journal of Anaesthesia 64: 537–541

Scrutton M 1997 Systemic opioid analgesia. In: Reynolds F (ed) Pain relief in labour. BMJ Publishing Group, London, ch 5

Sweet BR 1997 The pelvic floor and its injuries. In: Sweet BR, Tiran D (eds) Maye's midwifery: a textbook for midwives. Baillière Tindall, London, ch 32

Telfer FM 1997 Relief of pain in labour. In: Sweet BR, Tiran D (eds) Maye's midwifery: a textbook for midwives. Baillière Tindall, London, ch 32

Thibodeau GA 1990 Anthoney's textbook of anatomy and physiology, 13th edn. Times Mirror/Mosby College Publishing, St Louis

Thorp AJ, Breedlove G 1996 Epidural analgesia in labour: an evaluation of risks and benefits. Birth 23(2): 63–83

Thorp AJ, Nielson PE 1996 The effect of labour progress and the mode of delivery. Fetal and Maternal Medicine Review 8: 29–55

UKCC 1992 Standards for the administration of medicine. UKCC, London

UKCC 1998 Midwives rules and code of practice. UKCC, London

Wittels B 1990 Exogenous opioids in human breast milk: a preliminary study. Anaesthesiology 73: 864–869

9

Postnatal pain

Maureen Boyle

INTRODUCTION

Postnatal wards have long been known as the 'Cinderella service', often starved of staff and resources and becoming the area where it is most difficult to meet women's needs. Likewise, the puerperium is often undervalued, and although some research has been carried out into various aspects affecting the quality of women's experiences at this time, the amount is minimal compared to that directed towards the antenatal and labour periods.

The puerperium is also a time which many women feel least prepared for, and much of the research carried out around women's experiences after birth comment on how the amount of pain is generally a very unwelcome surprise. Postnatal pain is almost universal – in one study 95% of women reported at least one type of pain during the first postnatal day (Dewan et al 1993). At a time when a new mother needs to be at her fittest to cope with sleepless nights, rushed or missed meals and perhaps overwhelming emotional

131

demands, many women are also dealing with the debilitating effects of pain. Of course this pain, like any pain, may be perceived as worse by a woman who is physically and/or psychologically stressed – a description of many (or most) women after labour.

The shock of unexpected postnatal pain can even overshadow a fulfilling birth experience and the joy of a healthy newborn. A woman in pain may find it difficult to give her baby as much attention as she would wish – in a survey of 2000 women, many respondents felt a preoccupation with perineal problems which interfered with their relationship with their baby (Greenshields & Hulme 1993). The physical problems related to painful breasts/nipples and perinea mean women may find breastfeeding difficult, and may give up. Pain from abdominal or perineal wounds, or muscular pain, may cause lack of mobility which not only compromises a mother's ability to care for her baby and therefore may affect her confidence and self esteem, but also may result in dangerous physical effects such as deep vein thrombosis.

Studies into factors associated with postnatal depression have identified that it is not the 'quality' of the birth experience which is related, but the woman's feelings about it – unexpected interventions over which she has no control are strongly associated with the development of depression (Romito 1989). The presence of unexpected postnatal pain can therefore also be assumed to be a potential trigger for postnatal depression.

As well as specific therapies for different areas of pain, oral analgesia is a common treatment. Paracetamol has been shown to be the most commonly used oral analgesic on postnatal wards (Sleep & Grant 1988b). However many trials have found non-steroidal anti-inflammatory drugs (NSAIDs) such as mefenamic acid (Ponstan) more effective (Dewan et al 1993). Many other common oral analgesics used, such as co-codamol, contain codeine, and while these may be effective in relieving pain, they may also produce the unwanted side-effect of constipation.

Complementary therapies such as acupuncture, aromatherapy, homeo-pathy, etc. are gaining in popularity and many women find them effective. However most midwives are not trained in their use, and therefore are governed by professional regulations.

A survey by Dewan et al (1993) which looked at the types and timescale of reported postnatal pain, found that initially, in new mothers perineal pain was the most common site for pain (77%), and for multiparous women it was uterine cramps (77%). However by the fourth postnatal day, breast pain had increased for both breast- and bottle-feeding women, to involve the majority of women. Over this period 42% of women felt they had not achieved good pain relief. There is obviously much scope for an improved response to women's needs in the postnatal period.

PERINEAL PAIN

Although acute perineal pain, most commonly following trauma and sutures to the perineum, can complicate the early postnatal period, it is also a pain that can continue well into the puerperium – and longer – for many women. In a study carried out in 1984, Jennifer Sleep found 25% of women with perineal trauma had pain after 10 days, and 8% after 12 weeks (Sleep et al 1984). A more recent study found 32% of first-time mothers and 42% of multiparous women had perineal pain at 8 weeks, and 16% and 4% respectively at 12–18 weeks (Glazener et al 1993).

The scope of this problem was recognized in the National Childbirth Trust publication *The Perineum in Childbirth* (Greenshields & Hulme 1993). Interestingly, in their survey of more than 2000 women, it was noted that some women with intact perinea reported pain, whereas others with both an episiotomy plus tear did not. The point was also made that many women were told they were 'well healed' early in the postnatal period, and wondered why they continued to feel such pain. Scar tissue of course is not flexible, and may take many weeks – or months – to feel comfortable. The importance of the woman's feelings and perceptions needs to be paramount in the midwife's assessment and advice.

Apart from the obvious pain from a perineal wound, this may be compounded by infection, which may result in increased and prolonged pain. Another cause of severe and persistent perineal pain is the presence of a haematoma or abscess – careful examination may be necessary to diagnose these conditions, as they may be hidden, sited in the vaginal vault, although felt as perineal pain.

Many treatments have been identified for the perineum, with varying reports of success, although no one therapy will be effective for all women.

Although not strictly part of the postnatal period, a big influence on the pain, healing and long-term sequelae of perineal trauma is suture material and technique used. Subcuticular suturing has been demonstrated to cause less postnatal pain, and long-term dyspareunia may be related to the suture material used (Grant 1989). There is also some research suggesting that if selected second-degree tears are not sutured, they heal as well (or better) than those sutured. Women who were able to compare a previous experience of sutures, with a subsequent birth with an unsutured tear, reported more pain with sutures (Head 1993).

As with other forms of postnatal pain, oral analgesics are widely used as a treatment for perineal wounds, with paracetamol the usual drug (Sleep & Grant 1988b). However, NSAIDs are probably of more use because of their anti-inflammatory action. Diclofenac sodium (Voltarol) is an effective analgesic, with anti-inflammatory properties.

Women with perineal trauma are often prone to constipation, due to fear of defecation, so a codeine-based drug would seem unsuitable. However one study reported that paracetemol/codeine (co-codamol) was a more efficient analgesia, without causing constipation, when compared with paracetemol/dextropropoxyphene (co-proxamol) (Jacobson & Bertilson 1993).

The most common therapy for perineal pain is water, and there is evidence that most women find bathing helpful (Sleep & Grant 1988a). Research has indicated that cold sitz baths are more effective than warm, but this was restricted to the initial period after the birth. Cold baths also proved very unpopular with the women, which rather limits their use (Ramler & Roberts 1986).

If using baths shared by others, for example on a postnatal ward, there is a potential risk of infection (Caddow 1989). A shower would undoubtedly be more hygienic, but it is questionable whether it would be as effective as a relaxed 'soak'.

Bath additives have either been proved to be ineffective e.g. salt & savlon; (Sleep & Grant 1988a) or have not yet been comprehensively studied. There is some research on the use of lavender oil (Dale & Cornwell 1993), which showed some limited benefit. Other substances used as 'perineal soaks' on pads, such as comfrey leaf, lavender flower and calendula flowers (Lewis 1994) and witch hazel/glycerine (Spellacy 1965), have also been studied, however there is no evidence of reliable effectiveness. Arnica tablets are also used by many women to promote healing, although the cream should not be used on broken skin. There is no doubt many women get relief from complementary therapies and provided these treatments are directed by a recognized practitioner in the field, no harm should be caused.

Ice packs are also widely used for perineal pain. Cold therapy immediately after trauma causes vasoconstriction, thereby decreasing oedema and relieving pain. However, this effect is not helpful after 24 hours, as the cold, by restricting blood flow, can interfere with wound healing (Rhode & Barger 1990). The form of the ice therapy is also relevant, with large ice packs, especially used by mobile women, having the potential to cause ice burns on surrounding tissue.

In the past foam or rubber rings have seemed to provide comfort for women with perineal trauma when sitting, but these are no longer recommended because it was felt that the resulting impaired venous return could either predispose to thromboembolism, or the compression could increase oedema to the perineum and hence result in increased pain and delayed healing (Lowthian 1985). Nevertheless, women continue to use their own substitutes (e.g. children's swimming rings), which probably suggests they have a positive comfort value (Grant & Sleep 1989). A new innovation, the 'Valley cushion' has been developed to allow comfortable sitting for those with perineal trauma, but there is only limited information on its effectiveness at present (Yearwood 1991).

The use of hairdryers on a cool setting directed at the perineum is no longer advocated, as the resultant excessive drying can inhibit healing (Glossop 1996).

Research on a combination of local anaesthetic and steroid application (e.g. epifoam) has shown an increase in the number of wound breakdowns and inhibited wound healing (Greer & Cameron 1984). However local anaesthetic by itself, as a spray, cream or gel, has been shown to be effective in several trials (Grant & Sleep 1989), although it seems to be not much used (Sleep & Grant 1988b).

There is no evidence of ultrasound and pulsed electromagnetic energy treatment reducing pain (Sleep 1990).

On-going perineal pain is the most common reason for the non-resumption of sexual relations after birth. This aversion may become long-term abstinence, which can lead to the breakdown of the relationship (Comport 1990). Perineal pain therefore has the potential to cause the destruction of the family unit so newly created – its importance cannot be overemphasized.

BREAST AND NIPPLE PAIN

Breast and nipple pain is very common in the early postnatal period, with about 44% of new mothers and about 37% of multiparous women reporting moderate to severe pain on day 4 (Dewan et al 1993). Nipple trauma and engorgement can be interrelated, as nipple trauma may result in decreased feeding which in turn causes engorgement, or engorgement may lead to difficulty in getting the baby properly fixed on, causing nipple trauma. Because painful breasts and nipples are the main reason for giving up breastfeeding, it is an area of obvious importance for midwives.

The milk ejection ('let down') reflex, in response to the oxytocin release, is experienced by some women as a sharp pain. This can be a normal physiological occurrence in these women, and usually will pass off completely within a few moments, when feeding will become pain free. Nevertheless it can be a cause of distress for some women, and they will benefit from explanation and support from their midwives – some suggest using deep breathing practised for labour at this time.

The predominant cause of nipple pain or cracking is incorrect positioning of the baby (Woolridge 1986). Therefore, in the majority of cases, if positioning is corrected the nipple trauma will heal spontaneously (Inch & Renfrew 1989). Nevertheless, many forms of suggested treatments have evolved over the years.

There are many creams, gels and sprays on the market which purport to prevent/cure sore nipples, however there is no evidence that any preparation is effective (Inch & Renfrew 1989). Some substances, such as soap and alcohol, can actually increase nipple soreness (Royal College of Midwives 1991). Many midwives advise expressing colostrum or breast milk, and applying it to the damaged area – although there is no evidence as to its efficacy, it is extremely unlikely to do any harm, and may also in fact have a psychological benefit (Inch 1990). Limiting feeding does not help prevent nipple soreness (Carvalho et al 1984) and in fact may make matters worse by causing engorgement (Woolridge & Fisher 1988). Resting the nipple but expressing the milk may suppress lactation, as the prolactin response to artificial expressing is not as good as that obtained by the baby (Howie 1985). Nipple shields (either thick or thin) have not been shown to aid nipple healing (Nicholson 1985) and in addition have been shown to reduce the transfer of milk to the baby (Woolridge et al 1980) predisposing the woman to engorgement.

Apart from poor positioning of the baby, other causes for nipple soreness are few. Research has not shown that hair colour or skin type predisposes a woman to nipple trauma (Inch & Renfrew 1989). However nipple candidiasis (thrush) can cause nipple soreness as well as breast pain. There is a correlation between nipple candidiasis and maternal vaginal candidiasis, recent antibiotic use and baby's oral/perianal candidiasis (Tanquay et al 1994). Once diagnosed, treatment is a topical application to the nipple of oral antifungal medication after feeds for at least 3 weeks. If deep breast thrush is present the woman also needs oral treatment. The baby should also be treated for oral and perianal candidiasis (Saunders 1997).

Mastitis manifests as a red, painful, swollen area on the breast, usually limited to one lobe, and systemic symptoms such as pyrexia, tachycardia and generalized aches. Fifty per cent of lactating women with mastitis do not have an infection (Inch & Fisher 1995). Infective mastitis can be quickly diagnosed with a leucocyte and bacterial count from a specimen of milk, without waiting for bacterial cultures (Thomsen et al 1984). Non-infective mastitis can be treated by continuing to breastfeed, perhaps in combination with expressing (Thomsen et al 1984), whereas an infection needs antibiotics and milk to be expressed and discarded (Inch 1990). It is important to either keep feeding or expressing as a breast abscess is more likely if a woman with mastitis stops feeding (Marshall et al 1975). Pain from mastitis is usually treated according to the symptoms, with oral analgesia, antipyrexials and comfort measures such as warm compresses.

Engorgement of the breasts is a common cause of postnatal pain. In the first few days after birth, it may be due to the increased blood flow to the breasts, thereafter a 'milk engorgement' can be caused by insufficient emptying of the breast. It can generally be prevented by baby-led feeding without restriction, however some babies – premature, sick or babies sedated from drugs used in labour – may not cooperate.

Treatment for engorgement begins with encouragement of the baby to feed. Hot or cold compresses (or alternating the two) have long been advocated, but there is no research establishing its value (Inch & Renfrew 1989). The use of oxytocin to reduce engorgement has not been proved to be effective (Inch & Renfrew 1989).

Many midwives suggest that cabbage leaves applied to the breasts can relieve (or indeed, prevent) engorgement. A randomized controlled trial (Nikodem et al 1993) found more benefit felt by the 'cabbage leaf group', but it was not statistically significant. However, at 6 weeks, more women who received cabbage leaf treatment were likely to be breastfeeding. Although it was difficult to know if this was due to increased comfort earlier on, or increased attention from carers, it was still a positive finding.

Besides efforts to reduce the engorgement, women may also find paracetamol useful for pain relief.

Women who may almost inevitably suffer engorgement to some extent are those who choose not to breastfeed, or who deliver a stillbirth. Binding the breasts has been found to be effective in suppressing lactation, but not in treating engorgement (Brooten 1983). There is also some evidence that fluid restriction may reduce the symptoms of engorgement in those suppressing lactation (Parazzini et al 1989), but care would need to be taken to avoid adverse effects such as urinary tract infections, constipation, etc.

Bromocriptine has been commonly prescribed in the past for lactation suppression. In a study comparing it with breast binders, initially it appeared more successful, but when treatment stopped at 3 weeks, a 're-bound' effect showed, with all the women experiencing problems at this time from the bromocriptine group (Shapiro & Thomas 1984, Parazzini et al 1989). In addition, treatment with bromocriptine should be accompanied by careful monitoring of blood pressure in postnatal women – cases of hypertension, myocardial infarction, seizures or strokes and mental disorders have been reported in postnatal women given bromocriptine for lactation suppression (British Medical Association & Royal Pharmaceutical Society of Great Britain 1997). The United States Food & Drug Advisory Committee recommended that bromocriptine should not be used to treat breast engorgement in 1989, and has since moved to ban it for this use (Lancet News 1993).

AFTER-PAINS

The release of oxytocin from the posterior pituitary gland, especially in response to the baby breastfeeding, acts on the oxytocin receptors in the uterus, causing uterine cramps or 'after-pains'. These pains can range in degree from a mild 'period-type' discomfort to a severe pain, likened by the mother to contractions. After-pains often worsen with increased parity, and indeed some multiparous women may describe them as 'worse than labour'.

After-pains are very common, they are the most frequent (77%) pain reported following birth by multiparous women (Dewan et al 1993). Despite being so common, there is very little literature concerning after-pains, and most advice centres around oral analgesia (e.g. paracetamol) especially prior to feeding, hot water bottles and warm baths. Some women have also found using the breathing exercises learned for labour helpful when breastfeeding.

A pathological reason for after-pains is the uterus attempting to expel retained products, and this cause must always be considered.

POSTOPERATIVE PAIN

Although caesarean sections have become extremely safe over the past decades, there is still considerable morbidity associated with them (especially emergency caesarean sections) (Hillan 1995), including infection, increased need for blood transfusion and decreased mobility leading to further complications.

Pain is a complicating factor for all women post caesarean section; however finding the right way to treat this pain may be problematical. There is also a question as to how good midwives may be at accurately assessing pain. An American study of nurses and women following caesarean section showed nurses' and patients' assessment of pain differed considerably (Olden et al 1995).

The vast majority of women will receive opioid analgesia (e.g. morphine, diamorphine, pethidine) for at least a short time postoperatively. Traditionally this has been offered as an intramuscular injection, theoretically given at the patient's request, although in fact very often coinciding with the ward's drug rounds. This has the obvious disadvantage of a woman perhaps waiting in pain, because she knows 'they'll be around soon', or alternatively taking unnecessary analgesia when offered because it's convenient.

Reduced sedation and good pain relief is essential to achieve mobility. Morphine delivered intravenously via a PCA (patient-controlled analgesia) pump has been found to provide less sedation and greater satisfaction (Rayburn et al 1988). Epidural morphine infusions have also been shown to give good pain relief (Newman & Cashman 1993), and in a comparison with intramuscular papaveretum, increased mobility in the epidural diamorphine infusion group was demonstrated (Patrick et al 1991). However, potential side-effects such as respiratory depression mean careful observation needs to be made of these women, and continuous pulse oximetry monitoring has been suggested (Newman & Cashman 1993). Other side-effects of morphine/diamorphine include itching, urinary retention and nausea.

A continuous epidural infusion of bupivacaine (marcain) can be used and this has been demonstrated to provide a good pain relief, and also to improve breastfeeding. In one study women who received a continuous epidural infusion of bupivacaine had breastfed babies with greater weight gain than those in the control group (Hirose et al 1996). It is not known whether increased comfort made feeding easier, or whether the babies were less sedated and therefore fed better, however it was an interesting result.

Bupivacaine can also be delivered direct to the wound site by regular instillation via a catheter sited beneath the rectus sheath through the abdominal wound. In a study in which all women had PCAs of a morphine regimen, those that also received bupivacaine to the wound used less morphine and reported less nausea and sedation (Mecklem et al 1995).

Whatever opioid analgesic is used, adding a NSAID such as diclofenac (Voltarol) in suppository form to the regimen reduced the need for opioids, as there was less breakthrough pain (Newman & Cashman 1993).

BACKACHE

Postnatal backache is present in up to 44% of all women (Buggy & MacEvilly 1996). There is much controversy at present as to whether, or to what degree, new backache is associated with epidural use during labour (or with the drug regimen used in the epidural). Low back pain was reported on day 1 (53% of women who had had an epidural and 43% of those who did not) and at 6 weeks post delivery (14% vs 7%) by MacArthur & MacArthur (1995). The combination of epidural and short labour was said to increase the rate of postnatal backache by Clark & MacQueen (1993), and new long-term backache was found to be more common in those who used epidurals by Russell et al (1993).

It may be considered that epidural use is more common in those labours or deliveries which are prolonged or otherwise problematic, and therefore more likely to predispose to postnatal complications such as backache. However even after correcting for these cases, an increased rate of backache was seen in those using epidurals in a survey of more than 10 000 women. It was concluded that because there was no increase in backache following epidurals for elective caesarean sections, the most likely reason was the postural strain of labour with an epidural (MacArthur et al 1991).

Other more recent studies have not demonstrated an association between epidurals and new backache (Buggy & MacEvilly 1996, Russell et al 1996). It may be that the increased awareness of potential back problems with epidurals has made midwives more conscious of the dangers of postural strain, and this, together with the increased mobility present with new epidural drug regimens ('low dose' or 'mobile' epidurals using bupivacaine plus an opioid), have influenced these findings.

Other associations found with postnatal back pain include a previous history of back problems, younger age and increased weight (Breen et al 1994).

HEADACHE AND OTHER NEUROLOGICAL SYMPTOMS

Newly occurring long-term frequent headaches and/or migraines, within 3 months of delivery were present in about 4% of 10 000+ women surveyed by MacArthur et al (1991). A strong association was found in this study with epidural use, and with those who also suffered backache. Headaches not associated with epidurals occurred most frequently in young multiparous women, or following caesarean section with a general anaesthetic.

'Dural tap' headaches following accidental dural puncture during epidural insertion can be treated with an epidural blood patch, although this often does not immediately relieve the headache, and analgesia may continue to be needed. Saline infusion into the epidural space has not been shown to prevent postdural puncture headache (Shah 1993). Dural taps have been associated with new long-term headaches/migraines – in one group studied symptoms lasted from 9 weeks to 8 years (MacArthur et al 1993).

Other neurological symptoms such as increased dizziness or fainting, increased numbness or tingling in the lower back, buttocks or legs and visual disturbances (with migraines) were found to be more common following epidural use (MacArthur et al 1992, Tubridy & Redmond 1996). Weakness in the legs and tingling in feet and toes has been reported to be associated with forceps delivery (MacArthur et al 1991).

MUSCLE PAIN

Neck and shoulder pain is commonly associated with general anaesthetic (MacArthur et al 1991), but 24% of those who reported these symptoms had not received a general anaesthetic (Dewan et al 1993). It is not unreasonable that the rigours of labouring and giving birth may give rise to a transient painful neck and shoulders – tense shoulders are many women's response to stress. However this may be compounded by poor breastfeeding positions, and midwives should be ready to advise about postural strain while feeding.

SYMPHYSIS PUBIS DYSFUNCTION

Diastasis symphysis pubis is the separation of the symphysis as a result of the relaxation of the muscles and ligaments, and can happen antenatally, during labour or present as a new condition in the postnatal period. It is often associated with the use of the lithotomy position in the second stage. Pain can be mild to severe around the pubis, groin and thighs and may also be experienced in the lower back. Mobility is usually extremely compromised (Fry et al 1997).

Diagnosis is from symptoms or with pelvic X-ray or ultrasound (Cockshoot 1995). Treatment is analgesia and anti-inflammatory drugs and rest, and by referral to a physiotherapist who can supervise mobilization (perhaps with aids such as crutches) and provide other pain relief (e.g. TENS, hydrotherapy) as necessary. Complementary therapies may also be of help.

See Chapter 2 for a full description of symphysis pubis dysfunction.

URINARY TRACT SYMPTOMS

The bladder in the postnatal period is easily distensible and prone to incomplete emptying. This predisposes the woman to cystitis and ascending urinary tract infection. Problems with micturition are more common following operative deliveries and/or the use of an epidural, when catheterization (especially if repeated) is more common. Fifty per cent of patients with repeat catheterization develop bacteriurea (Dennis 1989). Urinary tract infections need to be speedily recognized and treated to prevent pain from these conditions.

Treatment of a diagnosed infection is with the appropriate antibiotics, but analgesia may be necessary for any pain, and increased fluid intake, especially of fluids such as cranberry juice, may be beneficial.

HAEMORRHOIDS

In a survey showing 18% of women reporting haemorrhoids postnatally, it was reported that only 16% of these had disappeared by 3 months (MacArthur et al 1991). An increase in occurrence and severity was also associated with increased parity.

It is important that these women do not become constipated, which will only worsen their situation. Advice should be given on fibre in the diet and fluid intake, and if necessary a bulk forming agent (e.g. Fybogel) is better than laxatives (Rush et al 1989). Haemorrhoid preparations come as suppositories or cream, and contain local anaesthetics to alleviate the pain, and corticosteroids to reduce inflammation. In severe cases when other treatment is unsuccessful, a referral to a gastrointestinal clinic for further treatment may become necessary.

CONCLUSION

Many surveys have emphasized the unexpectedness of postnatal pain – women expect pain in labour but are surprised to have painful symptoms afterwards. If the unexpectedness of postnatal pain is one component of its unpleasantness, and indeed its potential association with postnatal depression, perhaps there would be benefit from preparing women more completely. In a survey of patients undergoing surgery, those who were well prepared preoperatively on what to expect during recovery did better according to many criteria (Wallace 1984). However it would be a challenge for midwives to prepare women for all the potential areas of postnatal pain, without causing unnecessary anxiety and fear.

It has been noted that much of the research into methods of alleviating postnatal pain may be compromised by the human element (Grant & Sleep 1989). A sympathetic and attentive carer delivering an analgesic treatment may go a long way to relieving some of the common discomforts following childbirth, regardless of the treatment she dispenses. This, perhaps more than anything, demonstrates the value of the midwife's role in the postnatal period.

ANNOTATED BIBLIOGRAPHY

Chamberlain G, Wraight A, Steer P 1993 Pain and its relief in childbirth: the results of a national survey conducted by the National Birthday Trust. Churchill Livingstone, Edinburgh

The results and suggested implications from data collected from all deliveries in the UK during one week in June 1990, assessing pain in labour and analgesia. A report on the follow-up survey done at six weeks postnatal includes information on physical and mental health following delivery.

Greenshields W, Hulme H 1993 The perineum in childbirth: a survey of women's experiences and midwives' practices. National Childbirth Trust, London

A survey of mothers and midwives, undertaken by the NCT, into perineal trauma. Measures to promote healing and to relieve pain postnatally, as well as the long-term effects, are included.

MacArthur C, Lewis M, Knox E 1991 Health after childbirth: an investigation of long-term health problems beginning after childbirth in 11,701 women. HMSO, London

This book investigates the types and frequency of health problems that start after childbirth, and explores their possible determinants from many different social, obstetric and anaesthetic factors.

REFERENCES

Breen T, Ransil B, Groves P, Oriol N 1994 Factors associated with back pain after childbirth. Anesthesiology 81(Jul): 29–34

British Medical Association & Royal Pharmaceutical Society of Great Britain 1997 British National Formulary, no 33, March. Pharmaceutical Press, Oxon

Brooten D 1983 A comparison of four treatments to prevent and control pain and engorgement in non-nursing mothers. Nursing Research 32: 225–229

Buggy D, MacEvilly M 1996 Do epidurals cause back pain? British Journal of Hospital Medicine 56(2–3): 99–101

Caddow P 1989 Applied microbiology. Scutari, London

Carvalho M, Robertson S, Klaus M 1984 Does the duration and frequency of early breast feeding affect nipple pain? Birth 11: 82–84

Clarke V, McQueen M 1993 Factors influencing backache following epidural analgesia in labour. International Journal of Obstetric Anesthesia 2: 193–196

Cockshoot A 1995 Diastasis symphysis pubis – a painful problem. Changing Childbirth Update 4 Dec, 10

Comport M 1990 Surviving motherhood. Ashgrove Press, Bath

Dale A, Cornwell S 1993 The role of lavender oil in relieving perineal discomfort following childbirth: a blind randomized clinical trial. Journal of Advanced Nursing 19(Jan): 89–96

Dennis J 1989 The physiology of management of the puerperium. In: Turnbull A, Chamberlain G (eds) Obstetrics. Churchill Livingstone, Edinburgh, ch 6

Dewan G, Glazener C, Tunstall M 1993 Postnatal pain: a neglected area. British Journal of Midwifery 1(Jun): 63–66

Fry D, Hay-Smith J, Hough J et al 1997 Symphysis pubis dysfuntion. Midwives 110(1314): 172–173

Glazener C, Abdalla M, Russell I, Rempleton A 1993 Postnatal care: a survey of patients' experiences. British Medical Journal 1(2): 67–74

Glossop C 1996 Perineal care after childbirth. Health Visitor 69(3 Mar): 96–99

Grant A 1989 Repair of perineal trauma after childbirth. In: Chalmers I, Enkins M, Keirse M (eds) Effective care in pregnancy and childbirth. Oxford University Press, Oxford, ch 68

Grant A, Sleep J 1989 Reflief of perineal pain & discomfort after childbirth. In: Chalmers I, Enkins M, Keirse M (eds) Effective care in pregnancy and childbirth. Oxford University Press, Oxford, ch 79

Greenshields W, Hulme H 1993 In: Oliver S (ed) The perineum in childbirth. NCT, London

Greer I, Cameron A 1984 Topical pramoxine & hydrocortisone foam vs placebo in symptoms & wound healing. Scottish Medical Journal 29: 104–106

Head M 1993 Non-suturing of tears to the perineum. In: Proceedings of the International Confederation of Midwifery, 23rd International Congress, Vancouver, Canada, pp 809–822

Hillan E 1995 Postoperative morbidity following caesarean delivery. Journal of Advanced Nursing 22: 1035–1042

Hirose M, Hara Y, Hosokawa T, Tanaka Y 1996 The effect of postoperative analgesia with continuous epidural bupivacaine after cesarean section on the amount of breast feeding and infant weight. Anesthesia Analgesia 82: 1166–1169

Howie P 1985 Breastfeeding: a new understanding. Midwives Chronicle 98(1170): 184–192

Inch S 1990 Postnatal care relating to breast feeding. In: Alexander J, Levy V, Roch S (eds) Postnatal care: a research-based approach. Macmillan, London, ch 2

Inch S, Fisher C 1995 Mastitis: infection or inflammation? Practitioner 239(Aug): 472–476

Inch S, Renfrew M 1989 Common breastfeeding problems. In: Chalmers I, Enkins M, Keirse M (eds) Effective care in pregnancy and childbirth. Oxford University Press, Oxford, ch 81

Jacobson J, Bertilson S 1993 Analgesic efficacy of paracetamol/codeine and paracetamol/dextropropoxyphene in pain after episiotomy and ruptures in connection with childbirth. Journal of International Medical Research 15(2): 89–95

Lancet News 1993 Bromocriptine. Lancet 243(8872): 675

Lewis L 1994 Team time: using herbs to help heal the unsutured perineum. Midirs. Midwifery Digest 4: 455–456

Lowthian P 1985 A sore point. Nursing Mirror 161(9): 30–32

MacArthur C, Lewis M, Knox E 1991 Health after childbirth. HMSO, London

MacArthur C, Lewis M, Knox E 1992 Investigation of long term problems after obstetric epidural anaesthesia. British Medical Journal 304(6837): 1279–1282

MacArthur A, Lewis M, Knox E 1993 Accidental dural puncture in obstetric patients and long term symptoms. British Medical Journal 306(6882): 883–885

MacArthur A, MacArthur C 1995 Epidural anaesthesia and low back pain after delivery: a prospective cohort study. British Medical Journal 311(7016): 1336–1339

Marshall B, Happer J, Zirbel C 1975 Sporadic puerperal mastitis: an infection that need not interrupt lactation. Journal of American Medical Association 233: 1377–1379

Mecklem D, Humphrey M, Hicks R 1995 Efficacy of bupivacaine delivered by wound catheter for post-caesarean section analgesia. Australian and New Zealand Journal of Obstetrics and Gynaecology 35: 416–421

Newman P, Cashman J 1993 What's new in post delivery pain relief. Maternal and Child Health June: 170–174

Nicholson W 1985 Cracked nipples in breastfeeding mothers: a randomized trial of three methods of management. Nursing Mothers of Australia Newsletter 21: 7–10

Nikodem V, Danziger D, Gebka N, Gulmezoglu A, Hafmeyr G 1993 Do cabbage leaves prevent breast engorgement? A randomized controlled study. Birth 20(Jun): 61–64

Olden AJ, Jordan ET, Sakima NT, Grass JA 1995 Patients' versus nurses' assessments of pain and sedation after cesarean section. Journal of Obstetric, Gynecologic and Neonatal Nursing 24: 137–141

Parazzini F, Zanaboni F, Liberati A, Tognono G 1989 Relief of breast symptoms in women who are not breastfeeding. In: Chalmers I, Enkins M, Keirse M (eds) Effective care in pregnancy and childbirth. Oxford University Press, Oxford, ch 82

Patrick J et al 1991 A comparison of epidural diamorphine with intramuscular papaveretum following caesarean section. International Journal of Obstetric Anesthesia 1(Sept): 25–28

Ramler D, Roberts J 1986 A comparison of cold and warm sitz baths for relief of postpartum perineal pain. Journal of Obstetric, Gynaecologic and Neonatal Nursing 15: 471–474

Rayburn WF, Geranis BJ, Ramadei CA, Woods RE, Patil KD 1988 Patient-controlled analgesia for post-cesarean section pain. Obstetrics and Gynecology 72: 136–139

Rhode M, Barger M 1990 Perineal care, then and now. Journal of Nurse Midwifery 35: 220–230

Romito P 1989 Unhappiness after childbirth. In: Chalmers I, Enkins M, Keirse M (eds) Effective care in pregnancy and childbirth. Oxford University Press, Oxford, ch 86

Royal College of Midwives 1991 Successful breastfeeding, 2nd edn. Churchill Livingstone, Edinburgh

Rush J, Chalmbers I, Enkin M 1989 Care of the new mother. In: Chalmers I, Enkins M, Keirse M (eds) Effective care in pregnancy and childbirth. Oxford University Press, Oxford, ch 78

Russell R et al 1993 Assessing long term backache after childbirth. British Medical Journal 306(6888): 1299–1303

Russell R, Dundas R, Reynolds F 1996 Long term backache after childbirth: prospective search for causitive factors. British Medical Journal 312(7043): 1384–1388

Saunders S 1997 Breast pain in the lactating mother. Midwives 110(1308): 8–9

Shah J 1993 Epidural pressure during infusion of saline in the parturient. International Journal of Obstetric Anesthesia 2(Oct): 190–192

Shapiro A, Thomas L 1984 Efficacy of bromocriptine versus breast binders as inhibitors of post partum lactation. Southern Medical Journal 77: 719–721

Sleep J 1990 Postnatal perineal care. In: Alexander J, Levy V, Roch S (eds) Postnatal care: a research-based approach. Macmillan, London, ch 1

Sleep J, Grant A 1988a Salt in bathwater: a randomised controlled trial to compare the routine addition of salt or savlon bath concentrate during bathing in the immediate post-partum period. Research and the Midwife Proceedings, Manchester pp 65–75

Sleep J, Grant A 1988b Relief of perineal pain following childbirth: a survey of midwifery practice. Midwifery 4(Sept): 118–122

Sleep J, Grant A, Garcia J, Elbourne D, Spencer J, Chalmers I 1984 West Berkshire perineal management trial. British Medical Journal 189(6455): 587–590

Spellacy W 1965 A double-blind controlled study of a medicated pad for relief of episiotomy pain. American Journal of Obstetrics and Gynecology 92: 272

Tanquay K, McBean M, Jain E 1994 Nipple candidiasis among breastfeeding mothers. Canadian Family Physician 40: 1407–1413

Thomsen A, Espersen T, Maigaard S 1984 Course and treatment of milk stasis, non-infectious inflammation of the breast and infective mastitis in nursing women. American Journal of Obstetrics and Gynecology 149: 492–495

Tubridy N, Redmond J 1996 Neurological symptoms attributed to epidural analgesia in labor: an observational study of 7 cases. British Journal of Obstetrics & Gynaecology 103: 832–833

Woolridge M 1986 Aetiology of sore nipples. Midwifery 2: 172–176

Woolridge MW, Baum JD, Drewett RF 1980 Effect of a traditional and of a new nipple shield on sucking patterns and milk flow. Early Human Development 4: 357–364

Woolridge M, Fisher C 1988 Colic, 'overfeeding' and symptoms of malabsorption in the breastfed baby: a possible artefact of feeding. Lancet ii: 382–384

Wallace V 1984 Psychological preparation as a method of reducing the stress of surgery. Journal of Human Stress Summer: 62–77

Yearwood J 1991 The Valley Cushion. Midwives Chronicle 104(1246): 336

10

Fetal pain

Sarah Keeble

INTRODUCTION

This chapter poses a number of interesting questions, many of which are not easily answered, some of which provoke ethical debate.

Does a fetus feel pain and, if pain occurs, at what gestational age can it be felt? Are we talking about pain in the true sense of the word or are we talking about the ability to be able to perceive pain? Assuming that the fetus does feel pain, what are the implications for practice with regard to ethical issues such as termination of pregnancy and, for the diagnostic procedures that are currently carried out on the fetus, is adequate analgesia, sedation, used?

Before examining these questions in any great depth, it is important to look at the word 'pain' in a little more detail. There are many definitions:

Pain ... is a highly personal experience, depending on cultural learning, the meaning of the situation, and other factors that are unique to the individual (Melzack & Wall 1988).

Merskey in 1986 offered the following definition which was subsequently used by the International Association for the Study of Pain, Subcommittee on Taxonomy (1979).

> *Pain is an unpleasant sensory and emotional experience associated with actual or potential tissue damage, and described in terms of such damage.*

Note: pain is always subjective. Each individual learns the application of the word related to injury in early life. This definition combines both the physiological and psychological attributes of the pain experience. The latter definition talks about applying meaning to pain based on experiences in early life: how early? The question of fetal memory must surely arise here, and should we be more interested as health professionals in alleviating pain sensations in utero, thus eliminating this personal experience very early in life. The neonate would then have no recollections of any pain sensations from being in utero. Feeling pain or having an awareness of pain along with the issues surrounding the unborn infant's ability to recognize pain are all dependent on the development of the sensory pathways in the human fetus. A summary of this development along with clarification of terms such as 'awareness' and pain 'perception' follows.

THE DEVELOPMENT OF SENSORY PATHWAYS IN THE HUMAN FETUS

Being aware of pain and being able to feel and perceive pain are dependent upon structural and functional links between the cerebral cortex and other parts of the central and peripheral nervous system. Terms such as 'awareness' or 'perception' of pain are complicated phenomena and can be easily confused. To clarify this, Kupferman (1995) believe that awareness of a cortical phenomenon requires input from the higher centre of the brain. Over the years, research has proven that fetal awareness of pain is impossible until at least the stage that sensory connections first penetrate the cerebral cortex at around 26 weeks' gestation (Klimach & Cooke 1988). Even though the penetration of this sensory information is vital, it may still not be adequate for the actual perception of pain to take place (Royal College of Obstetricians and Gynaecologists 1997). The actual perception of pain requires further development and maturation of the nervous system as a whole and this continues well into infancy. This can be further clarified by McCaffery & Beebe (1994) who defined pain as:

> *Pain is whatever the experiencing person says it is, existing whenever the experiencing person says it does.*

This definition clearly cannot relate to neonates as they do not vocalize or localize nor have they learnt how to perceive their painful experiences. This is why the skills to assess neonatal pain are of paramount importance to the nurses caring for them as they are the neonates' advocate. Poor pain assessment leads to poor management and untreated pain in itself has detrimental consequences (see Ch. 11).

When considering the above, it would seem impossible to be able to make distinctions between pain awareness and pain perception in association with fetal life. However, by looking at sensory development, clarification regarding pain phenomena in relation to developing structures and gestational age can be sought.

It is important to look at the following structural developments in Box 10.1.

The skin

The awareness/perception of pain is a function of the sensory nervous system which starts peripherally with the skin (Fig. 10.1). Specialized sensory nerve endings are found throughout the tissues of the body: obviously, these nerve endings need to develop before they can fully function. These receptors are called nociceptors because they respond to noxious stimuli (pain, discomfort).

It is important to point out here that noxious stimuli can be divided into three categories:

◆ Mechanical changes to the nociceptor such as stretching or compression.
   ◆ Thermal changes – obviously heat or cold
   ◆ Chemical changes – commonly such chemicals are produced by the body in response to inflammatory changes. These chemicals include bradykinin, serotonin and proteolytic enzymes (Vander et al 1994).

Nociceptors are not divided into the three categories just mentioned: some respond to mechanical or thermal changes while others will react to all three. Humphrey (1978) reported that sensory development (pain receptors) of fetal skin begins early in the first trimester of pregnancy. Earlier studies by Gleiss & Stuttgen (1970) have shown that the density of cutaneous nociceptive nerve

---

Box 10.1 Outline of structural developments in the fetus

◆ Skin (sensory receptors)
   Reflex movements of the fetus
   Spinal cord connections
◆ Brain
   Thalamus
   Cortex

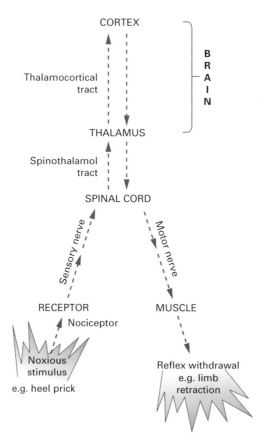

Figure 10.1 Pain pathway from the sensory nerve to the brain.

endings in the late fetus and newborn baby may equal or even exceed that of adult skin. This is interesting because if there are more nociceptors then surely as professionals we should be asking how much more analgesia can we safely give to these patients? We should not be giving the minimum of doses – surely more nociceptors means more pain! In 1964, Humphrey looked at the correlation between the appearance of human fetal reflexes and the development of the nervous system. This showed that cutaneous sensory perception appears in the perioral area of the human fetus in the seventh week of gestation and then gradually spreads to all other cutaneous and mucous surfaces by 20 weeks of gestation. From the perioral area, these nerve ends spread to the rest of the face, the palms of the hands, and the soles of the feet by the eleventh week, to the trunk and proximal parts of the arms and legs by the fifteenth week, reaching all mucous surfaces by the twentieth week (Valman & Pearson 1980). Payne et al (1991) stated that it is only after 28 weeks' gestation that nerve endings are seen near to the surface of the skin, prior to this they are largely subdermal or below the surface layer of the skin.

Reflex movements of the fetus

It is important at this stage to consider the reflex movements of the fetus as this is normal developmental behaviour and not necessarily related to noxious stimuli or pain.

As long ago as 1985, it was found that spontaneous fetal movements could be detected by ultrasound from 7.5–8 weeks' gestation (Prechtl 1985). Andrews & Fitzgerald (1994) found that reflex responses to noxious stimuli can be activated in preterm infants, as preterm as 23 weeks' gestational age. This study did, however, point out that although those responses to noxious stimuli could be evoked, their properties are different to the responses seen in adults. These differences include:

◆ The reflex responses in the fetus are larger in amplitude.
◆ The reflex responses are of longer duration.
◆ Non-noxious stimulation such as touch can cause a reflex response in the fetus and responses can be activated from a larger area of the body surface than adult reflexes.

From this, the Royal College of Obstetricians and Gynaecologists (1997) concluded that there are important differences in the reflex connections between the immature and adult spinal cords, thus making it more difficult to prove that a reflex movement is caused by noxious stimuli.

Spinal cord connections

In order for information to reach the central nervous system, there has to be connections with the peripheral nervous system. These connections are by means of sensory nerves. The nociceptor becomes the sensory nerve which needs to grow into the spinal cord, via the dorsal root, and to make connections with neurones in the dorsal part of the spinal cord. In the human fetus, the spread of cutaneous receptors is preceded by the development of synapses between the sensory nerve fibres and the interneurones in the dorsal horn of the spinal cord which first appear during the sixth week of gestation (Wozniak et al 1980, Okado 1981). Konstantinidov et al (1995) discussed how sensory fibres grow into the spinal cord at 14 weeks' gestation, they also pointed out that noxious information which is carried in C fibres terminates in the superficial parts of the spinal dorsal horn and at 19 weeks' gestation these still have not formed connections in the spinal cord. So it is non-noxious stimuli that are felt during and before 19 weeks and not noxious stimuli! Therefore, the time of onset of responses to painful stimuli is unknown, but according to Konstantinidov et al (1995) it is unlikely to be before 19 weeks' gestation. Two types of sensory nerve fibres carry pain signals: type A delta fibres and type C fibres. Anand & McGrath (1993) explain that C fibres are unmyelinated and A delta fibres are thinly myelinated which affects the transmission speed of painful stimuli to the spinal cord and brain. According to Guyton (1991), when properly developed type A delta fibres are capable of carrying messages at speeds of 6–30 m/s and type C fibres are around 12 times slower, carrying messages at around 0.5–2 m/s. This is where acute and chronic pain come in. Type A delta fibres carry the fast pain signals, acute pain, and type C carry slow chronic pain signals.

It is important at this point to briefly discuss myelination and its development. Lack of myelination has in the past been an issue around a lack of maturity in the neonatal nervous system (Tilney & Rosett 1931). This has been widely used in the argument that preterm or full-term neonates are not capable of feeling pain (Lippman et al 1976, Shaw 1982, Anand et al 1985, Hatch 1987). However, this is interesting; as previously mentioned, with peripheral nerves, nociceptive impulses are carried through unmyelinated C fibres and thinly myelinated A delta fibres (Schulte 1975, Anand & McGrath 1993). So where is the issue here; lack of myelination appears to be a very poor excuse considering nociceptive impulses are carried in unmyelinated and thinly myelinated fibres. According to Schulte (1968), incomplete myelination merely implies a slower conduction velocity in the nerves or central nerve tracts of neonates which is offset completely by the shorter interneurone and neuromuscular distances travelled by the impulse. Gilles et al (1983) highlighted that nociceptive nerve tracts in the spinal cord and central nervous system undergo complete myelination during the second and third trimesters of pregnancy. Pain pathways to the brain stem and thalamus are completely myelinated by 30 weeks' gestation. To complete this section it is necessary to point out the process of pain transmission from the spinal cord to the brain.

In the dorsal horns of the spinal cord, axon terminals of the primary sensory neurones transmit their pain messages to secondary neurones. It is these secondary neurones that cross the central area of the grey matter in the cord and form tracts known as spinothalamic tracts in the lateral portion of the white matter of the cord. These tracts run the length of the cord to the brain, ending in the thalamus (Vander et al 1994).

FETAL DEVELOPMENT OF THE BRAIN

The thalamus

The Royal College of Obstetricians & Gynaecologists (1997) have summarized development of the thalamus (Box 10.2). Khan et al (1994) also highlight that only 40% of the synaptic input of the thalamus is from sensory pathways arriving from the spinal cord, brain stem and retina. The other 60% is from the cortex in the form of descending connections and these do not reach the thalamus before 20–21 weeks' gestation. As Sherman & Guillery

(1996) point out, this is important because thalamic functions beyond a simple feedback or filter system are dependent on feedback from the cortex. The descending fibres will only transmit nerve impulses from cortex to thalamus and not thalamus to cortex.

Hasegawa et al (1992) stated that myelination first occurs in the thalamus at 25 weeks' gestation, which is well before myelination occurs in the cortex at 35 weeks' gestation.

In summary then, the thalamus begins to mature earlier than the cortex but its function beyond a simple relay system depends on connections with higher levels of the nervous system which do not begin before 22 weeks' gestation.

The cortex

If a fetus is to be aware of or perceive external stimuli then it is essential that the cortex is functional. According to Klimach et al (1988), relatively little is known about human cortical development but one vital fact is that thalamocortical connections necessary for good communication between the thalamus and cortex are first observed penetrating the frontal cortical plate at 26–34 weeks of gestation. This means that before such a time there is no sensory input to the cortex. According to Marin-Padilla (1983), development of the fetal cortex begins at 8 weeks' gestation and by 20 weeks each section of the cortex has 10^9 neurones. However, as previously mentioned, it is the timing of the thalamocortical connections that is important with regard to fetal development and an awareness of pain.

Box 10.2 Summary of thalamus development in gestational week stages

6 weeks	It is poorly developed
From 6 to 8 weeks	Differentiation begins with the three zones (ventricular, intermediate and mantle) distinguishable
From 10 to 14 weeks	Segregation of neurones into groups of nuclei begin and some neurones have grown dendrites
13–14 weeks	Synaptic contacts/connections for transmission between neurones are observed
From 14 to 16 weeks	Segregation continues, neurones are maturing and some multipolar neurones appear (Mojsilovic & Zecevic 1991)
15–20 weeks	A great increase in both the number and maturation of synapses but they do not begin to acquire the pattern and structure seen in adults until 20–21 weeks' gestation (Khan et al 1994)

Development, hence maturation, of the human cortex is a prolonged process and this depends on the sensory input acquired in late fetal life and following birth. At 34 weeks' gestation, new neurones are still being generated and synaptogenesis continues for 2 years post birth, stimulated by sensory experiences. According to Casey (1991), imaging studies emphasize that there is no single cortical area associated with a painful stimulus; many different cortical areas are activated when a stimulus is felt. Even in adult life, structural and functional development of the nervous system continues. At some time during this development, it can be said that awareness is possible: this time cannot be accurately identified but the quality of awareness and therefore perception becomes evident during pregnancy (Royal College of Obstetricians & Gynaecologists 1997).

Both fast and slow pain signals (acute and chronic) are carried via the spinothalamic tracts to the brain. However, they terminate in different areas. From an anatomical point of view, this is important as it explains how the human can differentiate between acute and chronic pain in later childhood. As previously mentioned, a painful stimulus triggers different areas of the cortex, not just one. C fibres and A delta fibres stimulate different areas, and it is these separate areas that differentiate or interpret the pain signals. The fast pain signals are relayed via the brain stem and thalamus to the somatosensory area of the cortex. Here the message can be interpreted with accuracy so a child can point to the part of the body where the original pain stimuli came from. By contrast, slow pain signals terminate over a wide area of the brain stem and thalamus in an area known as the reticular activating system. Chronic pain signals continually stimulate the reticular activating system, increasing the excitability of the brain and so this type of pain is difficult to localize, hence, resting and sleeping is more difficult with chronic pain as the brain is in a state of excitement as a result of the termination of the pain signal in this area (Vander et al 1994).

It has been necessary to dwell on the structural development of the human fetus in order to gain an understanding of painful stimuli and at what age it is physically possible for a fetus to have an awareness of pain.

From all the researched evidence described so far in this chapter, it can be summarized that the anatomical and physiological facts indicate that thalamocortical connections do not penetrate the cortical plate before 26 weeks' gestation. No matter what else is occurring, it is these connections that are vital for sensory input to reach the fetal brain and trigger 'pain'. Although the fetus may show reactions before this time it cannot be aware of sensory stimuli. As the Royal College of Obstetricians & Gynaecologists (1997) conclude, it is not possible for a fetus to be aware of painful events before 26 weeks' gestation but because of the uncertainty that can occur regarding actual gestational dates/age, it is good practice to consider fetal analgesia or sedation for major intrauterine procedures performed at or after

24 weeks' gestation. This removes the possibility of any sensory information reaching the cortex, any meaning painful or otherwise.

By looking in depth at the structural development of pathways necessary for pain message to be recognized, the question concerning 'at what age does the fetus feel pain?' has been clarified. The issue around actual awareness and the actual perception of painful stimuli has also been addressed.

TERMINATION OF PREGNANCY

Questions around termination and the fetus being able to feel such procedures have been fully answered by looking at the physiological development in utero. This subject is open to huge ethical and moral debates, the question now is how are terminations carried out and whether adequate sedation and/or analgesia are used, and perhaps more importantly, how can we as professionals in this field ensure that the appropriate analgesia is given for the appropriate gestational age of the fetus. The next part of this chapter will briefly summarize current practices and procedures.

To a certain extent, advocacy comes in here, upholding the rights of the fetus. What are these 'rights', the right not to feel noxious stimuli? As previously mentioned, the time of onset of responses to noxious stimuli is unknown but it is unlikely to be before 19 weeks' gestation, as the sensory fibres that carry the stimuli have not formed connections in the spinal cord before this time (Konstantinidov et al 1995). This brings us back to the very first question surrounding fetal growth, 'does a fetus even have rights?'. This has many answers depending on one's own individual beliefs and feelings, beliefs on whether a fetus is a 'life' from conception or from delivery. Whatever our beliefs may be, it is only human to wish that no pain should be felt during termination and invasive diagnostic procedures.

Terminations are carried out either medically or by surgical intervention. If surgical, they are usually carried out under general anaesthetic especially at gestations beyond 10 weeks. Medical terminations are usually carried out under maternal sedation and analgesia especially after 12 weeks. Terminations after 24 weeks are only permitted for serious fetal abnormality.

Medical termination

After 14 weeks of pregnancy, prostaglandins may be given to women in order to induce labour and terminate (Bennett 1994). By using these drugs, uterine contractions are started which cause the cervix to dilate resulting in miscarriage. This usually occurs within 24 hours. If there are retained products of pregnancy, the procedure is completed by surgical evacuation of the retained products which is carried out under general anaesthesia.

When pregnancies are brought to an end because of fetal abnormality after 21 weeks, the procedure which may be either medical or surgical is usually preceded by an injection of potassium chloride into the umbilical cord or fetal heart which stops the fetal heart beat (Report of Working Party on Termination of Pregnancy for Fetal Abnormality 1996).

An alternative method of stopping the fetal heart beat before terminating a pregnancy is to cut the umbilical cord, this is done following dilatation of the cervix and immediately before the onset of surgical evacuation of both the fetus and placenta. This procedure is carried out under general anaesthetic (Royal College of Obstetricians and Gynaecologists 1997).

Surgical termination

This is carried out by either of the following:

♦ Cervical dilatation and removal of fetus. Before 12–14 weeks, the fetus and products of conception are removed by suction through a cannula and fetal death is instantaneous. According to Bennett (1994), it is far more humane for mother and fetus to terminate a pregnancy that is in the second trimester by dilatation and evacuation. After 14 weeks, the uterine contents are removed and death of the fetus occurs usually within a few seconds.

♦ Hysterotomy (incision of the uterus). This is carried out for fetuses with abnormalities where vaginal delivery is impossible.

♦ Hysterectomy (removal of the uterus). This is only carried out for serious maternal conditions, for example, malignancy and is only for gestations below 24 weeks. Hysterectomy for maternal reasons but where the fetus is of a viable gestation is preceded by a caesarean delivery, which is far more humane for the fetus.

If one considers what has been discussed previously regarding the anatomical and physiological evidence, it would appear that the fetus being terminated prior to 24 weeks' gestation will be unable to feel pain as it is incapable of receiving any sensory input to the higher centres of the brain. The Royal College of Obstetricians & Gynaecologists (1997) therefore recommend that for terminations at 24 weeks or later, depending on the surgical procedure, that feticide (fetal death) should be carried out using a technique that stops the fetal heart rapidly, for example an injection of potassium chloride. An alternative is the use of an opioid premedication which should be given to the mother and then allowed time to cross the placenta and therefore build up in the fetus. In such incidences, the fetus is therefore sedated prior to the termination.

At this point it is worth briefly discussing the question 'Does the fetus/unborn baby feel pain during labour?' After 24–26 weeks' gestation, the fetus has the necessary structures in place to be able to feel pain. According to Moore (1993), maternal stress such as that induced by labour or any painful procedure has an adverse effect on the fetus and therefore effective pain relief is beneficial for both the mother and fetus. On the other hand, Irestedt (1993) goes on to say that the stress response is suppressed in the baby whose mother has received a general anaesthetic but is preserved if epidural anaesthesia is used. Ramsay & Lewis (1995) studied the effects of birth condition on infants' cortical response to stress and one of his findings showed that the effects of a non-optimal birth condition in otherwise healthy term infants continued for at least the first 6 months of life. It is interesting that the stress response measured in babies following labour and vaginal delivery is higher than in those following elective caesarean section.

Over the past few years various research studies have been carried out which examine the stress responses of the human fetus. Giannakoulopoulos et al (1994), for example, looked at fetal plasma cortical and beta-endorphin response to intrauterine needling. Here it was found that the fetus shows a similar hormonal response to that of neonates, older children and adults when exposed to noxious stimuli. Ward Platt et al (1989) say that endocrine and metabolic response to stress is evident from the mid trimester of fetal life. McCullagh (1996) focuses on the physiological issues in fetuses as young as 3 months' gestation, saying that existing knowledge does not enable us to say that such an immature fetus will experience an unpleasant sensation as this requires proof that the spinal cord and subcortical structures associated with such functions are operational.

Assessing fetal pain is a difficult task and currently there are no validated tools in use in clinical practice to make such an assessment easier. Assessing the varied movements that the fetus makes in response to noxious stimuli would perhaps be a useful method. This is an area that clearly requires further research.

DIAGNOSTIC PROCEDURES

These can either involve fetal contact or not.

◆ Diagnostic procedures not involving fetal contact are:
  – amniocentesis;
  – placental biopsy/chorion villus sampling;
  – fetal blood sampling from the umbilical cord;
  – fetoscopy (direct inspection of the fetal anatomy by passing a fine endoscope through the maternal abdominal wall – seldom used as ultrasound provides sufficient accurate information.

All of the above are performed with careful guidance using ultrasound, thus ensuring that the fetus is not touched. It is important to note here that the umbilical cord has no nerve supply, therefore sensation is not transmitted.

◆ Diagnostic procedures involving fetal contact are:
  – fetal blood sampling from the umbilical vein in fetal liver;
  – withdrawal of fluid from a cystic organ, e.g. bladder;
  – biopsy of fetal skin, liver, muscle, tumour.

In these instances, fetal analgesia/sedation is not normally given (Royal College of Obstetricians and Gynaecologists 1997).

Along with diagnostic procedures, there are also invasive therapeutic procedures; these are divided into two groups:

◆ open surgery;
◆ percutaneous procedures.

Rice & Harrison (1997) explain that 'open' surgery involves a major operation on the mother, allowing surgery directly on the fetus. This surgery is not yet carried out in the UK.

Percutaneous procedures are carried out with ultrasound guidance under local anaesthesia to the mother. Many of these procedures do not involve direct fetal contact and are usually carried out between 20 and 34 weeks' gestation (Royal College of Obstetricians & Gynaecologists 1997).

For percutaneous therapeutic procedures that do not involve direct fetal contact, such as fetal anaemia requiring a transfusion via the umbilical cord, then the fetus is not involved nor are any areas capable of feeling any sensation involved. For percutaneous therapeutic procedures that involve direct fetal contact, such as a transfusion into the intrahepatic umbilical vein of the fetus, then it is likely that the mother is sedated and has received a local anaesthetic. Therefore, the fetus may be sedated and immobile. For some procedures, however, fetal sedation may be detrimental as fetal movement may assist in some incidences. It is very easy to think that strong analgesia should be given to fetuses requiring invasive procedures, but the long-term effects of these drugs needs careful consideration. Aynsley-Green (1996) explains that because the fetal nervous system is changing rapidly due to maturation and alteration of neurotransmitter receptor numbers and function, it may be harmful to give opioids and risk the normal pattern of development. It is important, therefore, that in each case where there may be a need to administer a sedative, analgesic or anaesthetic drugs when performing intrauterine procedures, the balance of fetal pain and noxious stimuli, if gestationally possible, must be weighed up against the harmful effects of such drugs. Again, advocacy and the professional judgement of practitioners comes into focus here. One question in this chapter left for discussion is fetal memory. This is an area that still requires a lot of further research.

Lipsitt (1997) and Moscovitch (1984) suggested that newborns may have a much greater capacity for memory than was previously thought possible. This is old news but what have we learnt over the past few years? Back in

1957, Jones said that pain itself cannot be remembered even by adults, only the experiences associated with the pain can be recalled. Merskey (1970), however, thinks that the issue around memory is important, because it has been argued that memory is necessary for the maturation of pain perception. Long-term memory requires a functional limbic system (Squire 1986). These structures are well developed and functioning during the newborn period (Prechtl 1995).

The developmental changes required for memory and learning, for example synaptic and molecular changes, depend on brain plasticity which is known to be highest during late prenatal and neonatal periods (Bischot 1985, Will et al 1985). Early painful experiences, excluding early fetal growth, may be stored in an area of the brain that is not accessible to conscious recall (Osofsky 1976). Janoy (1971) has collected data that claims that adult neuroses or psychosomatic illnesses may have origins in painful memories acquired during infancy or even neonatal life. However, this has not been substantiated. It is interesting that little of this literature refers to fetal life. Thompson & Spencer (1966) do, however, talk about habituation. They demonstrated that when exposed to repeated stimuli, a fetus responds at first and then subsequently ignores it. This acts as a screening mechanism, allowing the fetus to respond to any new or changing stimuli and represents one of the most basic modes of learning. According to Leader et al (1984), habituation has been reported in human fetuses from 25 weeks' gestation.

There is some evidence that the fetus remembers the mother's diet from in utero (Hepper 1992). Babies born to mothers who ate spicy food before birth and plain food while in hospital, sucked less successfully than those born to mothers who maintained the same diet pre- and postnatally. There is a recognition here between certain flavours in the postnatal milk being familiar (Galef & Sherry 1973).

Fetal memory still poses many questions.

CONCLUSION

This chapter has discussed many questions regarding fetal pain. Many of these questions raise ethical debate. It is hoped that the facts have been summarized and indeed highlighted. In order to gain an understanding of the topic and in order to bring about clarity to many of the questions raised, it has been necessary to dwell on the anatomical and physiological structures. Without presenting these facts, the whole question 'does the fetus feel pain' is left unanswered. The research evidence clearly defines what structures required to feel pain develop at what gestational age. No matter what our personal beliefs may be, research clearly points out when all the necessary connections between the spinal cord and brain and the interconnections within the brain are developed and able to receive sensory input. Having an understanding of this development has helped put issues such as termination of pregnancy and fetal diagnostic procedures into some kind of perspective. It is very clear that fetal pain and the many issues surrounding this require further work.

> **Useful resources**
>
> Many anti-abortion groups have published and discussed the rights of the fetus; however, pain is not directly discussed in many, and if it is as far as resources are concerned, the usefulness of these publications is doubtful.

ANNOTATED BIBLIOGRAPHY

Care Online. Human Sentence Before Birth.
http://www.care.rg.uk/issus/fs/hs_cont.htm

A report by the Commission of Inquiry into fetal sentence (1996). Produced by Alpha Information Services Ltd for CARE. This really goes over a lot of what is already talked about in the chapter but has a different approach.

Fitzgerald M 1993 Development of pain pathways and mechanisms. In: Anand KJS, McGrath PJ (eds) Pain in neonates. Pain research and clinical management, vol. 5. Elsevier, ch 2

This is an excellent, very in-depth chapter, covering the development of pain pathways.

Anand KJS 1993 The applied physiology of pain. In: Anand KJS, McGrath PJ (eds) Pain in neonates. Pain research and clinical management, vol. 5. Elsevier, ch 3

This chapter looks in-depth at nociceptive stimuli not only in the peripheral venous system but also in many other areas of the body.

Sparshott M 1997. Pain, distress and the newborn baby. Blackwell Science, London, ch 3

This chapter offers a more simplistic view of the nervous system development. It highlights the important structural developments and the gestational age at which they occur.

Craig KD, Whitfield MF, Graunau RVE, Linton J, Hadjistavropoulous HD 1993 Pain in the preterm neonate: behavioural and physiological indices. Pain 52: 287–299

This article examines the behavioural and physiological effects of pain in both preterm and term infants. it highlights the effects of heel lancing, an invasive procedure that is frequently carried out in neonatal units.

REFERENCES

Andrews K, Fitzgerald M 1994 The cutaneous withdrawal reflex in human neonates: sensitization, receptive fields, and the effects of contralateral stimulation. Pain 56: 95–101

Anand KJS, McGrath PJ 1993 Pain in neonates. Pain research and clinical management, vol 5. Elsevier Science BV, Amsterdam

Anand KJS, Brown MJ, Bloom SR, Aynsley-Green A 1985 Studies on the hormonal regulation of fuel metabolism in the human newborn infant undergoing anaesthesia and surgery. Hormone Research 22: 115–128

Aynsley-Green A 1996 Pain and stress in infancy and childhood: where to now? Journal of Paediatric Anaesthesia 6: 167–172

Bennett P 1994 Fetal stress responses (letter). Lancet: 344(8922): 615

Bischot HJ 1985 Influence of developmental factors on imprinting. Advanced Behavioural Biology 28: 51–59

Casey KL 1991 Pain and central nervous disease: the central pain syndromes. Raven Press, New York

Galef BG, Sherry DF 1973 Mother's milk: a medium for transmission of cues reflecting the flavour of the mother's diet. Journal of Comparative and Physiological Psychology 83: 374–378

Giannakoulopoulos X, Sepulveda W, Kourtis P, Glover V, Fisk N 1994 Fetal plasma cortical and β-endorphin response to intrauterine needling. Lancet 344: 77–81

Gilles FJ, Shankle W, Dooling EC 1983 Myelinated tracts: growth patterns. In: Gilles FJ, Leviton A, Dooling EC (eds). The developing human brain: growth and epidermiologic neuropathology. John Wright, Boston, pp 117–183

Gleiss J, Stuttgen G 1970 Morphologic and functional development of the skin. In: Stave U (ed) Physiology of the perinatal period, vol 2. Appleton-Century-Crofts, New York, pp 889–906

Guyton AC 1991 Textbook of medical physiology. WB Saunders, Philadelphia

Hasegawa M, Houdou S, Mito T, Takashima S, Asanuma K, Ohno T 1992 Development of myelination in the human fetal and infant cerebrum: a myelin protein immunohistochemical study. Brain and Development 14: 1–6

Hatch DJ 1987 Analgesia in the neonate. British Medical Journal 294: 920

Hepper PG 1992 Fetal psychology: an embryonic science. In: Nisius J (ed) Fetal behaviour – developmental and perinatal aspects. Oxford University Press, Oxford, ch 11, pp 129–156

Humphrey T 1964 Some correlations between the appearance of human fetal reflexes and the development of the nervous system. Progress in Brain Research 4: 93–135

Humphrey T 1978 Function of the nervous system in prenatal life. In: Stave U (ed) Perinatal physiology. Plenum, New York, pp 651–683

International Association for the Study of Pain, Subcommittee on Taxonomy 1979 Pain terms: a list with definitions and notes on usage. Pain 6: 249–255

Irestadt L 1993 The effects of analgesia and anaesthesia on fetal and neonatal stress responses. In: Reynolds F (ed) Effects on the baby of maternal analgesia and anaesthesia. Saunders, London, pp 163–168

Janoy A 1971 The anatomy of mental illness. Putnam's Sons, New York

Jones E 1957 Pain. International Journal of Psychoanalysis 38: 255

Khan AA, Wadhwa S, Bijlani V 1994 Development of human lateral geniculate nucleus: an electron microscopic study. International Journal of Developmental Neuroscience 12: 661–672

Klimach VJ, Cooke RW 1988 Maturation of the neonatal somatosensory evoked response in preterm infants. Developmental Medicine and Child Neurology 30: 208–214

Konstantinidov AD, Silos-Santiago I, Flaris N, Snider WD 1995 Development of the primary afferent projection in human spinal cord. Journal of Comparative Neurology 354: 11–12

Kupferman I 1995 Cognition and the cortex. In: Kandel ER, Schwartz JH, Jessell TM (eds) Essentials of neurological science and behaviour. Appleton and Lange, Connecticut, pp 347–363

Leader LR, Baillie P, Martin B, Molteno C, Wynchank S 1984 Fetal responses to vibrotactile stimulation: a possible predictor of fetal and neonatal outcome. Australian and New Zealand Journal of Obstetrics and Gynaecology 24: 251–256

Lippman N, Nelson RJ, Emmanovilides GC, Diskin J, Thibeault DW 1976 Ligation of patent ductus arteriosus in premature infants. British Journal of Anaesthesia 48: 365–369

Lipsitt LP 1977 The study of sensory and learning processes of the newborn. Clinical Perinatology 4: 163–186

Marin-Padilla M 1983 Structural organisation of the human cerebral cortex prior to the appearance of the cortical plate. Anatomical Embryology 168: 21–40

McCaffery M, Beebe A 1994 Assessment. In: Latham J (ed) Pain – clinical manual for nursing practice. Mosby, London, pp 13–42

McCullagh P 1996 Determining fetal sentience. Hospital Update (editorial): 5–6

Melzack R, Wall P 1988 The challenge of pain, 3rd edn. Penguin Books, London

Merskey H 1970 On the development of pain. Headache 10: 116–123

Merskey H 1986 Clarification of chronic pain: descriptions of chronic pain syndromes and definitions of pain items. Pain. Supplement 3: 217

Mojsilovic J, Zecevic N 1991 Early development of the human thalamus: Golgi and Nissl study. Early Human Development 27: 119–144

Moore J 1993 The effects of analgesia and anaesthesia on the maternal stress response. In: Reynolds F (ed) Effects on the baby of maternal analgesia and anaesthesia. Saunders, London, pp 148–162

Moskovitch M 1984 Infant memory: its relation to normal and pathological memory in humans and other animals. Plenum Press, New York

Okado N 1981 Onset of synapse formation in the human spinal cord. Journal of Comparative Neurology 201: 211–219

Osofsky JD 1976 Neonatal characteristics and mother–infant interactions in two observational situations. Child Development 47: 1138–1147

Payne J, Middleton J, Fitzgerald M 1991 The pattern and timing of cutaneous hair follicle innervation in the rat pup and human fetus. Brain Research; Developmental Brain 173–182

Prechtl HF 1985 Ultrasound studies of human fetal behaviour. Early Human Development 12: 91–98

Ramsay DS, Lewis M 1995 The effects of birth condition on infants: cortisol response to stress. Paediatrics 95: 546–549

Report of Working Party on Termination of Pregnancy for Fetal Abnormality 1996 Royal College of Obstetricians and Gynaecologists, London, pp 15, 21 (abstract)

Rice HE, Harrison MR 1997 Open fetal surgery. In: Fisk NM, More KJ (eds) Fetal therapy: invasive and transplacental. Cambridge University Press, Cambridge 27–35

Royal College of Obstetricians and Gynaecologists 1997 Fetal awareness: report of a working party. RCOG, London

Schulte FJ 1968 In: Linneweh F (ed) Fortschritte der Paedologie, vol 2. Springer-Verlag, Berlin, pp 46–64

Schulte FJ 1975 Neurophysiological aspects of brain development. Mead Johnson Symposium of Perinatal Developmental Medicine 6: 38–47

Shaw EA 1982 Neonatal anaesthesia. Hospital Update 8: 423–434

Sherman SM, Guillery RW 1996 Functional organisation of thalamocortical relays. Journal of Neurophysiology 76: 1367–1396

Squire LR 1986 Mechanisms of memory. Science 232: 1612–1619

Thompson RF, Spencer WA 1966 Habituation: a model phenomenon for the study of neuronal substrates of behaviour. Psychological Review 73: 16–43

Tilney F, Rosett J 1931 The value of brain lipoids as an index of brain development. Bulletin of the Neurological Institute, New York 1: 28–71

Valman HB, Pearson JF 1980 What he feels. British Medical Journal 280: 233–236

Vander AJ, Sherman JH, Luciano DS 1994 Human physiology, 6th edn. McGraw-Hill, New York

Ward Platt MP, Anand KJS, Aynsley-Green A 1989 The ontogeny of the metabolic and endocrine stress response in the human fetus, neonate and child. Intensive Care Medicine 15: 44–45

Will B, Schmitt P, Dalrymple-Alford J 1985 Brain plasticity, learning and memory: historical background and conceptual perspectives. Advanced Behavioural Biology 28: 1–11

Wozniak W, O'Rahilly R, Olszewskia B 1980 The fine structure of the spinal cord in human embryos and early fetuses. Journal für Hirnforschung 21: 101–124

11

Neonatal pain and its management

Raewyn Twaddle

KEY ISSUES

- ◆ Untreated pain
    - Short term
    - Long term
- ◆ Fetal pain
- ◆ Pain assessment
    - Chemical response
    - Behavioural responses
    - Physiological responses
- ◆ Difficulty with pain assessment
    - Infant behavioural state
    - Pain and agitation
    - Time
    - Attitudes
    - Lack of pain tools
    - Risks of opioids
- ◆ Pain assessment tools
    - NIPS
    - DSVNI
    - The neonatal pain assessment tool
- ◆ Pain management
- ◆ Comfort measures
    - Non-nutritive sucking
    - Sucrose
    - Swaddling, containment and nesting

INTRODUCTION

Due to technological advancement, and the development of neonatal intensive care units, neonates are now surviving very premature births. In the last decade there has been great progress made in the treatment of neonates, resulting in improved survival. However, this progress has been slower in the area of neonatal pain assessment and management, which lags well behind that of children and adults.

The undertreatment of pain in neonates, in the past, was a result of several myths that have since been dispelled. It was thought that neonates do not feel pain because:

◆ Neonates have unmyelinated pain fibres making the transfer of painful stimuli impossible (Gardner 1993).
◆ Objective pain assessment is impossible (Gardner 1993).
◆ Neonates do not have the ability to remember a painful event.
◆ Neonates are unable to communicate their pain.
◆ Analgesics and anaesthetics cannot be safely administered (Gardner 1993).

These views led to the widespread belief that neonates cannot feel pain. This resulted in surgery and other invasive procedures taking place without anaesthetic or analgesia. Through research it is now known that neonates have the ability to perceive pain (Anand & Hickey 1987), therefore the importance of understanding the effects of pain on neonates cannot be underestimated.

All healthy newborn infants undergo routine blood sampling usually via a heel prick. Fifteen per cent of these healthy newborns have an additional two to five heel pricks in the first week of life (Ramenghi et al 1996). Sick and premature infants require a much greater amount of invasive therapy. Porter (1989) estimates that sick infants undergo between 50 and 132 bedside procedures, every 24 hours. Many of these procedures are painful and are regularly performed without analgesia. Therefore it is important for the carer to ensure that blood tests are clustered where possible to reduce the painful procedures the infant has to endure.

It is now recognized that neonates have the ability to perceive pain. It is also possible to safely administer anaesthetics and analgesics in the neonate. There are many adverse effects of untreated pain in the fragile newborn. It is therefore extremely important for those caring for neonates to be able to accurately identify signs and symptoms of pain and know how to manage and evaluate the pain.

UNTREATED PAIN

Short term

There is an initial instability and behavioural reaction during, and for a short time after, a painful event. However, many less obvious reactions occur when an infant is in pain.

Infants cannot continue to react to pain for long periods without becoming exhausted. They then shut out stimulus and appear drowsy or fall asleep (Sparshott 1996). There is an absence of crying, often even in the presence of further painful stimuli. There may be a lack of eye contact or a fixed staring gaze. The infant may be limp and unresponsive. An infant in pain will have an altered sleep pattern. There are prolonged periods of rapid eye movement sleep (Marshall et al 1980). Sleep–wake cycles may become disturbed. Ninety per cent of infants undergoing circumcision without anaesthetic had disrupted behavioural states for more than 22 hours compared with 16% of uncircumcised infants (Marshall et al 1980). These behavioural changes make it very difficult to assess pain. The infant appears immobile and resting quietly as stress hormones have been depleted (Franck 1993).

Long term

The shut-out behaviour where the infant fails to make eye contact or respond to stimuli may interfere with parent–infant bonding. It may have an effect on their adaptation to the postnatal environment. Feeding behaviours may take longer to develop (Anand & Hickey 1987).

The persistent behavioural changes after circumcision imply that an infant has some memory of the event; a memory of painful experiences increases the infant's sensitivity to subsequent painful encounters. Taddio et al (1994) found that infants who were circumcised without anaesthetic had a higher pain score and cried longer when having their vaccinations 4–6 months later. The amount and frequency of painful stimuli could result in a permanent alteration in cerebral neuroanatomy (Franck 1993). Research on animals suggests that pain and stress in the neonatal period can influence adult behaviour.

FETAL PAIN

With the issue of neonatal pain receiving considerable attention, the question next asked is at what age can neonates perceive pain. No one is sure when parts of the fetal brain become mature enough to register pain. This is because of the very complex nature of pain perception. However, it is thought to be before 24 weeks of gestational age (Anand & Hickey 1987), i.e. before the age of legal viability.

Very prematurely born infants respond to painful stimuli (Anand & Hickey 1987, Craig et al 1993). The pain response involves the same behavioural and physiological changes as for full-term infants, i.e. alteration in facial expression, body movement and physiological parameters, although these changes are more subtle and less frequent than for full-term infants. This is thought to be because of the immaturity of the motor and central nervous systems. It may also be because of the fragility of the infant, as very premature infants are usually less physiologically stable.

Fitzgerald et al (1988) found preterm infants to have increased sensitivity to painful stimuli when compared to the full-term infants or adults. This would imply an even greater need for analgesia for this age group.

After birth the elements of the central nervous system required to transmit pain continue to mature and become more organized. While developing, the central nervous system is vulnerable to environmental influences. It may also be altered by external events, resulting in abnormal structural and functional development (Duffy et al 1984).

PAIN ASSESSMENT

There are many factors to consider when assessing pain. In older children and adults we depend on the individual's ability to perceive painful stimuli and then communicate that knowledge to us. The verbal communication of pain is the most reliable indicator of the degree of pain (McCaffey & Beebe 1989). Because neonates are preverbal their pain perception can only be surmised. The assessment of pain in neonates involves interpreting the non-verbal signs and behaviours displayed in response to painful stimuli. Once accurately interpreted prompt, safe and effective relief can be provided.

There is no single behaviour or group of responses that accurately or reliably indicates pain, therefore a multidimensional approach must be used. Pain can be assessed using three criteria: noting the infant's chemical or metabolic responses, observing the behavioural response and monitoring the physiological response.

Chemical response

The body's chemical response to pain is shown by alterations in hormonal and metabolic substrates. It provides objective data, but is impractical in the clinical situation because of costly and timely laboratory work and blood sampling.

Adults undergoing surgery showed an increase in stress hormones in response to tissue injury. The stress hormones included catecholamines – mainly adrenaline and noradrenaline – (Griesan et al 1985, Anand 1986), corticosteroids (Grunar et al 1981), growth hormone and glucagon (Anand et al 1985). An increase in stress hormones leads to the breakdown of fat, protein and carbohydrate stores (Anand & Carr 1989), which leads to an increase in blood ketone bodies. The suppression of insulin secretion leads to hyperglycaemia.

Neonates display this same response to tissue injury. However, the response duration is shorter but the metabolic changes are three to five times greater than in adults (Anand 1986). The accelerated stress response in neonates results in a great loss of already limited fat, protein and carbohydrate stores (Anand 1990).

The stress response is not so apparent when anaesthetics are used. The infants remain more clinically stable during surgery. There are also fewer postoperative complications when compared to those infants who have only minimal or no anaesthetic.

Behavioural responses

The changes in behaviour occurring in response to painful stimuli include cry, facial expression and body movement. Observations of these behavioural changes are frequently used by nurses to assess an infant's level of pain (Pozanki 1976). The changes in facial expression and body movement are many and varied. Not all neonates display the same changes. However, there are some changes that occur more frequently, and these are used for pain assessment. Because of the immaturity of the motor system the infant's limited repertoire of responses is displayed for a variety of reasons. The responses specific to pain must be isolated from hunger, stress and other non-noxious stimuli (Franck 1987a).

Cry

Crying is the neonate's primary method of communicating and is therefore an obvious indicator of pain. It is possible to distinguish a pain cry from other cries (Johnston 1989), such as hunger or fear. A pain cry is high pitched, harsh, shrill, tense and dysharmonic with higher peak frequencies (Levine & Gordon 1982). Crying in relation to pain has bouts of longer duration, with shorter intervals between cries and with more frequent vocalization (Porter et al 1986).

Although crying is an obvious and definite indicator of pain, it is not possible to determine the degree of pain the infant is experiencing. It is a common means of assessing pain by nurses (Franck 1987a), but it has some drawbacks. Crying cannot be used to assess pain in the ventilated infant. Very sick infants may not be able to muster a vigorous enough response to cry, which does not mean that they are not experiencing pain. An infant's ability to cry will be altered by drugs such as sedation or paralysing agents.

Facial expression

Neonates display the same pattern of facial expressions in response to painful stimuli as adults (Craig et al 1992). The most frequently occurring expressions are brow bulge, eye squeeze, deepening of the nasolabial furrow, open lips (Craig et al 1993, Stevens et al 1993), taut cupped tongue, brow lowering, horizontal stretch mouth and vertical stretch mouth (Craig et al 1993).

Neonates of all gestational ages display changes in facial expression in response to painful stimuli. However, there are fewer changes in the very preterm infant. The infant under 28 weeks' gestation at birth displays little response above baseline levels. This may be due to their very limited energy reserves, i.e. all the energy is directed towards maintaining survival. Full-term infants give a more vigorous facial expression to painful stimuli.

Motor response

Due to the immaturity of the motor system, a neonate's behavioural responses are generalized. Detailed research has come up with a response pattern which is unique to acute pain. The diffuse gross motor movements displayed in response to pain stimuli are most frequent during the most invasive portion of the procedure. This is the case for infants of all gestational ages, although infants of a younger gestational age display fewer motor movements (Craig et al 1993).

The motor response to acute pain incorporates body tension, position of the limbs and the presence of startling or trembling (Dale 1986). The torso and limbs are rigid (Johnston & Strada 1986) with extension and tension of the limbs. The initial body tension is followed by a residual rigidity, flexion and occasional thrashing of the limbs until a gradual recovery and return to baseline activity (Van Cleve et al 1995). The most frequently observed motor responses are flexed legs and arms, diffuse squirming and hand to face motions.

A healthy term infant will display vigorous gross motor movement as above, but a premature or sick infant may display a much reduced response (Grunau et al 1990) or become limp and flaccid (Jones 1989). This is probably due to the immaturity of the motor system and the limited energy reserves of the very sick infant. In a study by Fitzgerald & McIntosh (1989) preterm infants appeared to be more sensitive to painful stimuli than term infants.

Assessment of pain is made difficult by infants demonstrating the same repertoire of responses to a variety of different stresses. There is a wide variety of motor responses made in response to painful stimuli but very few are consistent with all infants. There also does not appear to be any consistency between infants of the same gestational age or weight (Van Cleve et al 1995).

Physiological responses

The physiological responses to pain in newborn infants are less predictable than in adults because of the immaturity of their autoregulatory systems. Assessing physiological responses to pain can be used. The response is consistent throughout the gestational ages (Craig et al 1993) and it is an easy means of assessment as monitoring equipment is usually in place in the neonatal intensive care unit.

The changes seen in response to painful stimuli are many. The heart rate and blood pressure increase and remain elevated after a procedure (Anand 1987). The administration of local anaesthetic prior to circumcision was reported to prevent alterations in heart rate and blood pressure (Williamson & Williamson 1983). Respiration may be increased or decreased. There is a period of suppressed respiration, i.e. breath holding (Craig et al 1993).

Often there is a very dramatic reduction in oxygen saturation levels (Van Cleve et al 1995). The decrease in oxygen saturation levels is especially apparent when a more vigorous motor response is provoked. It is likely that the fall in oxygen saturation levels is a response to being disturbed rather than to pain (Craig et al 1993).

Palmar sweating occurs in response to painful stimuli and it is accurate at indicating the degree of pain (Gedaly-Duff 1989). However, the palmar sweat glands mature around 37 weeks' gestational age (Harpin & Rutter 1982), which makes it an unsuitable measure for preterm infants.

An infant's colour often changes from pink to red. Hiccups and gasps are often observed (Van Cleve et al 1995). Peripheral temperature decreases, leaving a widening of the toe/core gap.

Overall the physiological changes, especially those in heart rate, blood pressure and oxygen saturations, result in a decreased perfusion of vital organs (Anand & Carr 1989) and alterations in intracranial pressure (Stevens et al 1993). As a result untreated pain may lead to an increased morbidity and mortality (Anand & Hickey 1987).

DIFFICULTY WITH PAIN ASSESSMENT

In the absence of a verbal response, pain assessment must use a multidimensional approach. In neonates this approach uses observation of the infant's behavioural and physiological responses to painful stimuli. Because of the relative immaturity of the neonate the responses shown to painful stimuli are not well defined and are therefore open to misinterpretation. In addition, there are many other factors that make pain assessment of the neonate difficult.

Infant behavioural state

An infant's state will range from deep sleep to vigorous alert crying. The response to painful stimuli will vary depending on which state the infant is in at the time of the procedure. Infants who are awake and attentive but inactive show the strongest behavioural response to painful stimuli. A procedure performed on an infant, initially in deep sleep, will elicit a less vigorous behavioural response. It is therefore likely that this infant will receive a lower pain score when assessed. This difficulty also arises in infants being sedated, i.e. artificially kept in a quieter state. The sedation drugs will interfere with the infant's behavioural response and may alter the pain assessment.

There are some infants who are too ill or stressed to respond to painful stimuli. This does not necessarily mean they do not feel pain, but they may be unable to respond due to the inability of the immature central nervous system to withstand stress (Frank 1993). It is known that nurses judge a more vigorous response to indicate more intense pain (Shapiro 1991). Therefore the more fragile sick infant is likely to receive a lower pain score. These are the infants most likely exposed to frequent painful stimuli.

Pain and agitation

Pain responses are very similar to agitation in neonates. The limited repertoire of behaviours available to the neonate means that the same behaviours are used for pain and agitation. In order to treat the infant every effort must be made to determine the cause of the behaviour. It is also important to remember that it is normal for infants to have periods of fussy unsettled behaviour.

Time

There are few behaviours displayed by all infants in response to painful stimuli. Yet, individual infants tend to repeatedly use the same behaviours. It is then necessary to spend a lot of time observing the infant to determine their individual pain response. Because of the demands on a nurse's time, not enough time is spent at the bedside to accurately assess pain (Gorski 1984). Caretakers are likely to recognize the individual's particular pattern of response if they know the infant well. This is especially important in preterm infants, as their response to painful stimuli is much reduced when compared to full-term infants. Therefore only a very sensitive judge or someone familiar with the infant would be able to determine the signs of distress (Craig et al 1993).

Attitudes

Anyone assessing and treating pain brings to the assessment their own attitudes and beliefs about pain. It has been found that nurses assessing pain are influenced by the patient's social class, ethnicity, age, sex and medical diagnosis (Cohen 1980). It has also been found that a higher pain score may be given depending on the nurse's own experience of pain and/or whose children have experienced severe pain (Burokas 1985).

The nurse's level of training and number of pain courses attended since registration has been shown to influence neonatal pain assessment (Page & Halvorson 1991). Knowledge of pain responses and the priority given to pain recognition and relief will determine the degree of successful assessment. Lack of knowledge and negative attitudes result in undertreatment of pain.

Lack of pain tools

The absence of pain tools suitable for assessing neonates has in the past hampered pain assessment. Without a means of objective assessment nurses are left trying to justify their assessment. It is difficult to defend an assessment without objective data. Franck (1987b) found that analgesics were used in less than half the situations when the nurse believed clinical signs indicated the need.

The absence of a pain assessment tool means there is inconsistency in pain assessment between nurses.

Risks of opioids

There is an increased risk of side-effects, especially respiratory, when using opioid analgesia on neonates. The undertreatment of pain is often rationalized, with concerns that the risks of giving analgesia outweigh any benefits for very sick neonates. It has been demonstrated that analgesia can be safely administered to the neonatal age group. It has also been shown that untreated pain increases morbidity and mortality in neonates.

In practice it has taken some time for attitudes and prescribing practices to change. By 1995, almost all anaesthetists believed that neonates of all gestational ages felt pain (De Lima et al 1996).

PAIN ASSESSMENT TOOLS

When assessing pain in neonates, the nurse must interpret the various behavioural and physiological responses displayed by the infant. When an objective pain tool is used for the assessment, the assessor's own attitudes and beliefs, i.e. biases, are reduced (see Box 11.1).

Pain assessment tools have been used successfully with adults and children. Only recently have they been used in neonates. The pain assessment tools cannot be used in isolation for neonates, as many other factors influence how a neonate will respond to painful stimuli. The environment, maturation of the central nervous system, state of alertness, duration and type of pain, drugs and the infant's general health (Lawrence et al 1993) all affect an infant's pain response. Every effort must be made to identify sources of pain, observe behavioural and physiological changes and take into account these additional factors to accurately assess the level of pain.

NIPS

The neonatal infant pain scale (NIPS) was developed by the Children's Hospital of Eastern Ontario. The NIPS incorporates facial expression, cry, breathing, arm movements, leg movements and state of arousal, for assessment. Each item from the scale has a score of 0, or 1, except cry which has a 0, 1 or 2 score. A score is given for each item at 1-minute intervals, before, during and after the painful procedure. Then a total score is given, with 7 being the maximum score for each minute.

Box 11.1 Pain assessment tools

◆ Provide a means for objective assessment
◆ Provide consistency between assessors
◆ Provide objective information to back up the nurses judgement
◆ Allow documentation of pain behaviour
◆ Provide a framework from which evaluation of pain relief can be measured

The NIPS was designed for acute pain stimuli during venous, capillary or arterial puncture. The scale does allow the assessor to determine the intensity of the pain response (Lawrence et al 1993) as it gives a score for each minute. The NIPS has been validated. It seems to be more consistent than the VAS score and shows no difference between assessors (Lawrence et al 1993). The NIPS provides an objective pain tool that can also be used to evaluate the effects of pain relief measures.

DSVNI

The Distress Scale for Ventilated Newborn Infants (DSVNI) uses the words pain and distress interchangeably. The scale assesses the physiological and behavioural responses of the ventilated newborn infant to pain and distress. The scale assesses changes in facial expression, body movement and colour, and observes changes in heart rate, blood pressure, oxygenation and temperature differential (Sparshott 1996). Facial expression and body movement have a score of 0–3 and colour 0–2. Physiological responses are collected only from monitored infants but are not scored. The significance of the physiological parameters is in their change from baseline levels which is then taken into account with the behavioural changes.

At least four assessments should be made, one before the procedure to provide a baseline level. A second assessment should be made during the procedure and two following the procedure. It is recommended that the third assessment is made 3 minutes after the procedure, and a final assessment at 1 hour following the procedure. This is to evaluate any pain-relief measures given. The aim is for the final score to be 0. The DSVNI does indicate the degree of pain or distress of the infant. Although the DSVNI is designed for ventilated newborns, there is no reason why it cannot be used for any neonate undergoing a traumatic procedure.

The neonatal pain assessment tool

This tool assesses facial expression, body movement, cry and physiological changes. For an accurate pain score all four categories must be assessed. Each category is given a score of 0 to 2, except for cry which is scored as 0 or 2. A maximum score would be 8 (Table 11.1).

PAIN MANAGEMENT

The aim of pain management is to minimize the adverse effects of pain. When the chemical response is reduced there is less breakdown of fat, protein and carbohydrate stores. A reduced behavioural and physiological

Table 11.1 NEONATAL PAIN ASSESSMENT TOOL   Up to 4 weeks' or 44 weeks' gestation

	Score	Description
Facial expression	0	Relaxed *neutral expression* *peaceful*
	1	Grimace *frown* *tongue protrusion* *chin quiver* *brow bulge (brow lowered* *and drawn together)* *pursed lips* *facial twitch*
	2	Severe grimace *eye squeeze (eyes closed* *and skin wrinkled)* *wide open mouth exposing gums* *taut tongue (pulled back into* *mouth)*
Body movement/ behaviour	0	Settled *uninhibited movement*
	1	Restlessness *fussing* *finger splaying* *squirming* *fisting* *gagging* *opening of bowels* *hiccough* *tension and twitching of* *extremities*
	2	Body tension *rigid posture* *trembling* *lying still with flexion/extension* *of arms/legs* *drawing knees up* *withdrawal* *startling*
Physiology (Accurate while implementing minimal handling)	2	Pain free *parameters within patients'* *own baseline*

Table 11.1 *Cont'd*		
	I	Mild pain *decreased SaO$_2$* *colour change (pale, dusky,* *grey around lips, mottled)* *gradual increase in HR, resp.* *and BP*
	2	Severe pain *palmar sweating* *increased blood sugars* *sudden increase in HR, resp.* *and BP* *gradual increase in number* *of bradycardic* *episodes*
Cry (Does not have to be audible)	0	Not crying
	2	Vigorous crying *rapid onset* *long duration cry* *tears*

Pain score above 2, give analgesia. Copyright: Keeble and Twaddle, August, 1995.

response will limit the reduction of oxygen to the tissues. In limiting the adverse effects of pain, the ability of the infant to cope with the painful experience will be maximized. Giving pain relief reduces the physiological instability, metabolic stress and behavioural responses produced by the painful stimuli. There is however a large difference between the analgesics and anaesthetics given to adults compared to infants. This is especially true of opioids. There is no doubt that analgesics should always be given to an infant in pain, as the physiological and metabolic instability caused by the stress responses increases morbidity and mortality (Anand & Hickey 1987). However opioids are often not given because of physicians' attitudes and beliefs towards neonatal pain.

Paracetamol is widely and safely used for mild pain. Oral absorption in the neonate is variable due to altered gastric emptying times. Gastric emptying is dependent on the maturity of the gastrointestinal system and there may be a deficiency in pancreatic enzymes.

Non-steroidal anti inflammatory drugs (NSAIDs) are not recommended for use in the neonatal period (British Medical Association and the Royal

Pharmaceutical Society of Great Britain 1996). They are gaining in popularity, with 11% of anaesthetists using NSAIDs for surgical pain (De Lima et al 1996). Mild opioids such as codeine can be used and work particularly well when combined with paracetamol. They do however have the same side-effects as strong opioids but seem to be well tolerated.

Strong opioids such as morphine and fentanyl work well. Side-effects, particularly respiratory, are seen more frequently in neonates. This is because of the immaturity of the excretory systems, particularly the renal system. It is also a result of the increased permeability of the blood–brain barrier.

The half-life of strong opioids is longer and more variable in neonates, with a range of 15–28 hours (Colditz 1991). With individual neonates showing a wide variability in their sensitivity to strong opioids their tolerance of the drugs cannot be predicted. The excretion of opioids can be further delayed in critically ill neonates. The variability of drug effect in neonates means that toxic accumulation of the drug can occur. Effects can be seen in some individuals receiving an amount considered desirable for others (Mainous 1995). Adverse reactions with strong opioids are more frequently seen when using large doses, frequent dosing intervals or with a rapid rate of administration (Farrington et al 1993).

Local anaesthetics have been successfully used, but again neonates are more susceptible to systemic absorption and therefore toxicity.

Topical anaesthetics may be absorbed systemically because of the thin layer of skin in neonates. Topical absorption is altered by the hydration and integrity of the skin.

COMFORT MEASURES

Nurses caring for neonates are not limited to the use of drugs to provide pain relief. There are many soothing strategies that can be employed to comfort an infant in pain or distress. These comfort measures are inadequate by themselves but are useful in conjunction with medication. Comfort measures may be effective only during one period of development and different strategies may work for different individuals. Soothing strategies such as non-nutritive sucking, swaddling, massage, containment and rocking reduce the behavioural responses to painful stimuli. These measures help the infant to gain organization, relaxation, general comfort and sleep (Shapiro 1989).

Non-nutritive sucking

Non-nutritive sucking may make use of the infant's fingers or hands or a pacifier to suck without nutritional benefit. Non-nutritive sucking has been shown to reduce the behavioural response to pain (Field & Goldson 1984). It was found to reduce the length of time crying and increased the quiet alert behaviour after heel prick and circumcision (Field & Goldson 1984). This is important, as it reduces the physiological instability caused by crying and vigorous motor movement.

Non-nutritive sucking seems to be a more effective comfort measure in the neonatal period than at 2 months of age (Campos 1989). The physiological response to pain does not seem to be reduced with non-nutritive sucking (Campos 1989).

Sucrose

Concentrated sucrose solution (25–50%) given immediately before a painful procedure reduces the length of time crying during the procedure. There is also a reduction in heart rate 3 minutes after a heel prick. When pain was assessed with a pain tool there was a reduced pain score at 3 minutes after the procedure (Ramenghi et al 1996).

Swaddling, containment and nesting

These comfort measures involve fixing the infant's limbs close to the body in a flexed position. Swaddling uses a sheet or blanket, containment involves the carer's hands and nesting uses the infant's bedding to ensure limbs are flexed close to the body. These measures decrease gross motor movements evoked in response to pain (Campos 1989). These measures may work by stimulating a variety of sensory channels such as thermal, tactile and proprioceptive. Swaddling does seem to be more effective in the 2-month-old age group (Campos 1989).

CONCLUSION

Studies have demonstrated the improved growth and development of infants when stimuli in the neonatal intensive care unit such as light, noise and handling are controlled. The need is now recognized to reduce other frequent and intense stress in the neonatal environment such as pain.

Pain provokes a stress response, altering the body's physiological and metabolic parameters, leading to increased morbidity and mortality. Although neonates are preverbal, their pain is communicated in their behavioural responses. These behavioural responses can be assessed and prompt pain relief given. Pain assessment is made difficult by the diversity and non-specific nature of the neonate's behavioural responses. Using a pain tool eliminates some of the assessor's unintentional biases.

Drugs for pain relief can be given safely, but they are less well tolerated and have more frequent side-effects than in other children and adults.

Pain left untreated has many serious long-term outcomes for the neonate that are only just being realized.

ANNOTATED BIBLIOGRAPHY

Crawford D, Morris M 1994 Neonatal nursing. Chapman & Hall, London, pp 295–308

Chapter 16 of this textbook discusses neonatal pharmacology. It looks at the absorption, metabolism and excretion of drugs in the neonate.

Mander R 1998 Pain and its control. Blackwell Science, Oxford, pp 195–202

Chapter 11 addresses the issues in relation to fetal and neonatal pain in particular pathophysiology, ethical issues, clinical application and debate. It is a very readable chapter, giving food for thought.

Merenstein G, Gardner S 1993 Handbook of neonatal intensive care, 3rd edn. Mosby Yearbook, London, pp 564–688

This chapter explains neonatal behavioural development, outlines infant states and provides explanations for behaviours in the neonatal intensive care unit.

Porter F, Wolf C, Gold J, Lotsoff D, Miller P 1997 Pain and pain management in newborn infants: a survey of physicians and nurses. Pediatrics 100(4): 626–631

This article looks at the knowledge and attitudes of physicians and nurses to neonatal pain. Despite believing that neonates regularly feel pain, they also believe that drugs or comfort measures are not given to provide adequate pain relief.

Twycross A, Moriarty A, Betts T 1998 Paediatric pain management: a multidisciplinary approach. Radcliffe Medical Press, Oxon, pp 77–94

This is an excellent text discussing pediatric pain. Chapter 6 broadly discusses pain assessment in the preverbal child.

Yeh TF 1991 Neonatal therapeutics, 2nd edn. Mosby Yearbook, London, pp 1–15, 375–386

Chapter 1 discusses pharmacokinetics of drug therapy in the neonate. Chapter 27 looks at the drugs commonly used in the neonate for medical, surgical and radiologic procedures.

REFERENCES

Anand KJS 1986 Hormonal and metabolic functions of neonates and infants undergoing surgery. Current Opinions in Cardiology 1: 681–689

Anand KJS 1990 Neonatal stress responses to anaethesia and surgery. Clinics in Perinatology 17: 207–214

Anand KJS, Carr DB 1989 The neuroanatomy, neurophysiology and neurochemistry of pain, stress and analgesia in newborns and children. Pediatric Clinics of North America 36: 795–822

Anand KJS, Hickey PR 1987 Pain and its effects in the human neonate and fetus. New England Journal of Medicine 317: 1321–1329

Anand KJS, Brown MJ, Bloom SR, Aynsley-Green A 1985 Studies on the hormonal regulation of fuel metabolism in the human newborn infant undergoing anaesthesia and surgery. Hormone Research 22: 115–128

British Medical Association and the Royal Pharmaceutical Society of Great Britain 1996 British National Formulary, no 28. Pharmaceutical Press, London

Burokas L 1985 Factors affecting nurses' decisions to medicate paediatric patients after surgery. Heart and Lung 14: 373–379

Campos R 1989 Soothing pain-elicited distress in infants with swaddling and pacifiers. Child Development 60: 781–792

Cohen FL 1980 Post surgical pain relief: patients' status and nurses' medication choices. Pain 9: 265–274

Colditz PB 1991 Management of pain in the newborn infant. Paediatric Child Health 27: 11–15

Craig KD, Prkachin KM, Grunau RVE 1992 The facial expression of pain. In: Turk DC, Melzack R (eds) The handbook of pain assessment. Guilford, New York, pp 257–276

Craig K, Whitfield M, Grunau R, Linton J, Hadjistavropoulos H 1993 Pain in the preterm neonate: behavioural and physiological indices. Pain 52: 287–299

Dale JC 1986 A multinational study of infant responses to painful stimuli. Paediatric Nursing 12(1): 27–31

De Lima J, Lloyd-Thomas A, Howard R, Summer E, Quinn T 1996 Infant and neonatal pain: anaesthetists perspectives and prescribing patterns. British Medical Journal 313: 787

Duffy FH, Mower G, Jensen F, Als H 1984 Neural plasticity: a new frontier for infant development. In: Fitzgerald HE, Lester BM, Yogman MW (eds) Theory and research in behavioural pediatrics, vol 2. Plenum, New York, pp 67–69

Farrington EA, McGuinness GA, Johnson GF, Erenberg A, Leff RD 1993 Continuous intravenous morphine infusion in post operative newborn infants. American Journal of Perinatology 10(1): 84–87

Field T, Goldson E 1984 Pacifying effects of non-nutritive sucking on term and pre-term neonates during heel stick procedures. Pediatarics 74: 1012–1015

Fitzgerald M, MacIntosh N 1989 Pain and analgesia in the newborn. Archives of Disease in Childhood 64: 441–443

Fitzgerald M, Millard C, MacIntosh N 1988 Hyperalgesia in premature infants. Lancet i: 292

Franck LS 1987a A national survey of the assessment and treatment of pain and agitation in The Neonatal Intensive Care Unit. Journal of Obstetric, Gynecologic and Neonatal Nursing 16: 387–393

Franck LS 1987b Pain in the non-verbal patient: advocating for the critically ill neonates. Pediatric Nursing 5(1): 65–68

Franck LS 1993 Identification, management and prevention of pain in the neonate. In: Kenner C, Brueggemeyer A, Porter Gunderson L Comprehensive neonatal nursing – a physiologic perspective. Harcourt Brace, Philadelphia, ch 40, pp 913–925

Gardner SL 1993 Pain and pain relief. In: Merenstein GB, Gardner SL (eds) Handbook of neonatal intensive care, 3rd edn. Mosby Year Book, St Louis, pp 496–502

Gedaly-Duff V 1989 Palmar sweat index use with children in pain research. Journal of Pediatric Nursing 4(1): 3–8

Gorski P 1984 Experiences following premature birth: stresses and opportunities for infants, parents and professionals. In: Call JD, Galenson E, Tyson RL (eds) Frontiers of infant psychiatry. Basic Books, New York, pp 145–151

Greisen G, Frederiksen PS, Hertel J, Christensen NJ 1985 Catecholamine response to chest physiotherapy and endotracheal suctioning in preterm infants. Acta Paediatrica Scandinavica 74: 525–529

Grunau RE, Johnston CC, Craig KD 1990 Neonatal facial and cry responses to invasive and non-invasive procedures. Pain 42: 295–305

Grunar MR, Fisch RO, Korsvik S, Donhowe JM 1981 The effects of circumcision on serum cortisol and behavior. Psychoneuroendocrinology 6: 269–275

Harpin VA, Rutter N 1982 Development of emotional sweating in the newborn infant. Archives of Disease in Childhood 57: 691–695

Johnston CC 1989 Pain assessment and management in infants. Pediatrics 16: 16–25

Johnston CC, Strada M 1986 Acute pain responses: a multidimensional description. Pain 24: 373–382

Jones MA 1989 Identifying signs that nurses interpret as indicating pain in newborns. Pediatric Nursing 15(1): 76–79

Lawrence J, Alcock D, McGrath P, Kay J, Brock MacMurray S, Dulberg C 1993 The development of a tool to assess neonatal pain. Neonatal Network 12(6): 59–66

Levine JD, Gordon NC 1982 Pain in prelingual children and its evaluation by pain induced vocalization. Pain 18: 85–93

Mainous R 1995 Research utilization: pharmacologic management of neonatal pain. Neonatal Network 14(4): 71–74

Marshall RE, Stratton WC, Moore JA, Boxerman SB 1980 Circumcision. Effects on newborn behavior. Infant Behavioral Development 3: 1–14

McCaffey M, Beebe A 1989 Pain clinical management for nursing practice. CV Mosby, Boston

Page GG, Halvorson M 1991 Pediatric nurses: the assessment and control of pain in preverbal infants. Journal of Pediatric Nursing 6(2): 99–106

Porter E 1989 Pain in the newborn. Clinics in Perinatology 16(2): 549–564

Porter F, Miller R, Marshall R 1986 Neonatal pain cries: effect of circumcision on acoustic features and perceived urgency. Child Development 57: 790–802

Pozanki EO 1976 Children's reactions to pain: a psychiatrists perspective. Clinical Pediatrics 15: 1114–1119

Ramenghi LA, Griffith GC, Wood CM, Levene MI 1996 Effect of non-sucrose tasting solution on neonatal heel-prick responses. Archives of Disease in Childhood 74: F129–F131

Shapiro C 1989 Pain in the neonate. Neonatal Network 8(1): 7

Shapiro CR 1991 Nurses judgements of pain intensity in term and preterm newborns. Journal of Pain and Symptom Management 6: 148

Sparshott MM 1996 The development of a clinical distress scale for ventilated newborn infants: identification of pain and distress based on validated behavioral scores. Journal of Neonatal Nursing April: 5–11

Stevens BJ, Johnston CC, Horton L 1993 Multidimensional pain assessment in premature neonates: a pilot study. Journal of Obstetric, Gynecologic and Neonatal Nursing 22(6): 531–540

Taddio A, Goldbach M, Ipp M, Stevens B, Karen G 1994 Effect of neonatal circumcision on pain responses during vaccination in boys. Lancet 345: 291–292

Van Cleve L, Johnson L, Andrews S, Hawkins S, Newbold J 1995 Pain responses of hospitalized neonates to venipuncture. Neonatal Network 14(6): 31–36

Williamson PS, Williamson RN 1983 Physiologic stress reduction by a local anaesthetic during newborn circumcision. Pediatrics 71(1): 36–40

Appendix
Physiology illustrations

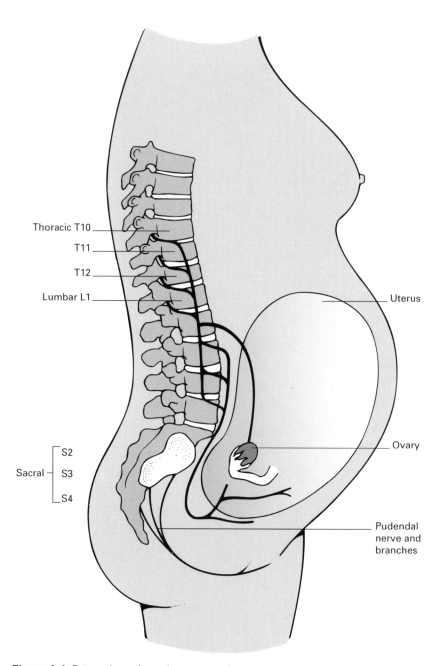

Figure A.1 Pain pathway from the spine to the uterus.

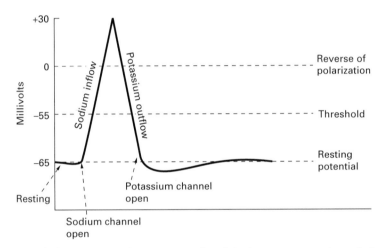

Figure A.2 Action potential in a neurone. Fast firing increases transmitter discharge therefore more pain is caused.

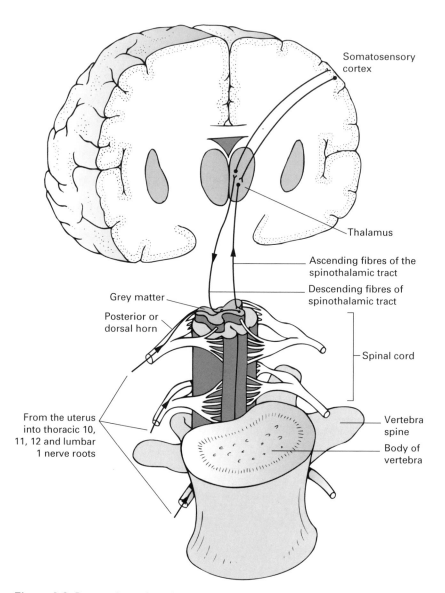

Figure A.3 Brain and spinal cord connections.

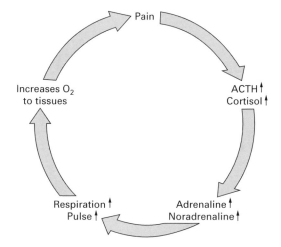

Figure A.4 Homeostasis in labour.

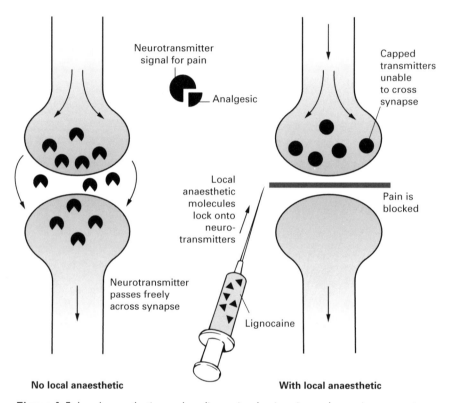

Neurotransmitter
signal for pain

Analgesic

Capped
transmitters
unable
to cross
synapse

Local
anaesthetic
molecules
lock onto
neuro-
transmitters

Pain is
blocked

Neurotransmitter
passes freely
across synapse

Lignocaine

No local anaesthetic

With local anaesthetic

Figure A.5 Local anaesthetics, such as lignocaine, bupivacaine and procaine, prevent transmission of pain in the sensory nerves by blocking the action potential and thus stopping pain transmission.

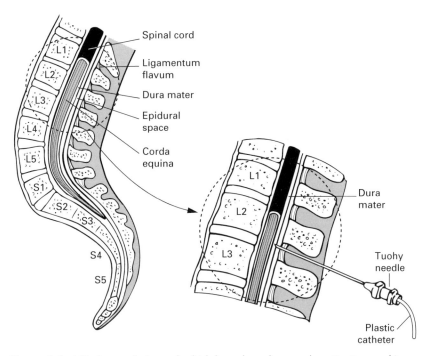

Figure A.6 A Tuohy needle is used, which has a large bore and centimetre markings to give a guide to the depth reached. Skill is needed to find the space between the ligamentum flavum and the dura mater.

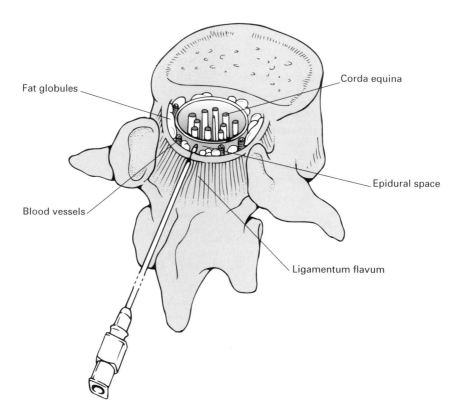

Fat globules

Corda equina

Epidural space

Blood vessels

Ligamentum flavum

Figure A.7 Needle positioned in the epidural space.

Index